SAFFRON WALDEN
in old photographs

H.C.STACEY

SAFFRON WALDEN
in old photographs

The C. W. Daniel Company Limited
Saffron Walden

First published in Great Britain
by The C. W. Daniel Company Limited
1 Church Path, Saffron Walden, Essex

© H. C. Stacey 1980

ISBN 0 85207 148 5

Printed in Great Britain by the
White Crescent Press Ltd, Crescent Road, Luton, Beds

Contents

Introduction

I look back and count myself fortunate that, on leaving school in June 1916 at the age of 14, I went to work, for 3s 6d a week, in the offices of Turner Collin & William Adams, solicitors at 14 Church Street.

Law clerks were expected then to write a good copperplate hand and I came under the influence of Arthur Raymer, another clerk, from Wenden. He spent most of his dinner hour turning up the Old Manorial Court Rolls and other documents to study the handwriting and texting, to enthuse over when I returned to the office. Raymer, the best penman in Saffron Walden then or since, not only taught me handwriting, texting and map drawing on parchment but, in the process, introduced me to some of Walden's history in those beautifully written records, The old law clerks who shared this interest in handwriting, *engrossing* we called it, have all passed on except for Miss Eva Scales who will recall days when writing, not typing, earned our bread and butter.

As my knowledge of the bricks and mortar of the town grew so did my interest in the people.

In 1929 I was invited to succeed Mr Henry Cox of the Town Clerk's department. Apart from being close to town affairs I found myself amongst all the muniments, at that time uncatalogued, unindexed and in a dirty state in the Town Hall strong room. They had been there, little disturbed, since 1879 when George Staccy Gibson included a strong room in his new Town Hall. What a challenge!

Then aged 27, enthusiastic, and in a fresh job concerning Walden, I made myself familiar with this Pandora's Box of records whenever time permitted. Turning out the Town Clerk's cupboard to familiarise myself with the contents I found *A Short History of the Members & Officials of the Corporation* compiled by Town Clerk J. G. Bellingham and extended by Charles Reed for a few years before putting to one side and forgetting.

When I talked to my chief about bringing it up to date he was encouraging and recounted events and people from his own experience. Mr Land and Mr Reed were also happy to satisfy my eagerness to learn what was what.

I wrote scores of letters begging photographs and tracing descendants. The time came, in 1934, when Mr Adams could invite members of the Council to meet the donors and to receive portraits of all but seven Mayors over the period 1835–1934. In later years I was able to reduce the number missing to three, Robert Paul (1838), C. B. Wilkins (1839) and Hannibal Dunn (1843). *The Members & Officers* record has been much extended since 1932.

In the early part of the Second World War the vicar, Dr L. Hughes, nervous about incendiary bombs being dropped on the church, asked the Council to remove all the Corporation records stored in the Muniments room over the south porch. The papers were packed in tea chests and taken to the Municipal Offices strong room where they remained until after the war. Their move led to a research into the history of Walden never before undertaken.

At this time I was Borough Food Officer and Councillor C. B. Rowntree was Chairman of my Food Control Committee. Mr Rowntree was respectfully referred to by those of us who worked with him, as C. B. R. and I will continue to do so here.

At one stage of food rationing expectant mothers could obtain extra milk on presentation of appropriate coupons obtainable at the Milk Office opposite the strong room. C. B. R. was one of the two staff manning the Milk Office and, as there were few applicants and as C. B. R. was not a man to sit and idle, he spent time examining the contents of the tea chests. Occasionally he came to my room to show me papers he had found, explaining what they were about and sometimes asking questions. In their move many bundles had come apart and sometimes C. B. R. had to turn out a whole box and meticulously sort loose papers into appropriate bundles. This was only a time filler and it was not until after the war that C. B. R. could give adequate time to study all the papers.

His discovery of papers relating to the Food Riots of 1795 and the murder of Walden's Chief Constable, William Campling, in 1849 stand out clearest in my memory. C. B. R. was a Rotarian and he gave talks to his club of these finds.

When he attended Almshouse Meetings he interested the trustees in the records relating to their own charity. I have always understood that it was the Rotary Club and the Almshouse Trustees who eventually persuaded C. B. R. to write a local history. They each offered £25 towards the cost of publication and C. B. R. was able to pay back this money from sales made.

During the time C. B. R. was Mayor and Chairman of the Housing Committee, he used to call on me daily and was a most conscientious Councillor. Sometimes he would consult me on subjects about which he was writing, and often I could help by producing records from the strong room. So started, for me, five or six years close association with C. B. R. and I was privileged to be his labourer. Councillor Hubert Collar, museum curator, was brought into the consultations too, and from the two of them I learned how essential it was, if one wrote history, to present facts and not introduce fiction.

After the war and up to 1950, I copied or abstracted numerous records, in my spare time to relieve C. B. R. of time-consuming chores so that he could devote himself to the writing of what became *Saffron Walden, Then & Now*. I was a frequent caller at 7 Springhill Road to leave or collect something, and my assistant, Miss Dyer, often found the time to do typing work for C. B. R.

When his book was finished C. B. R. talked to me about the clearing up he had to do and said he proposed to put all the various photographs and material into a brown paper scrapbook. I persuaded him to let me ask an old school pal of mine, Bert Cornell, who was a bookbinder, to make a book worthy of its purpose. Bert willingly agreed, I paid for the materials used and C. B. R. was delighted with the finished result. In it he pasted pages and illustrations from *Then & Now* and his surplus photographs used up about half the book. I added my own pictures and since that first book was filled 25 years ago Bert has made me four others. After all these years I will express again my appreciation to him for making the books.

David Campbell, Michael Haselgrove, Jack Lee and George Oakes all helped C. B. R. with pictures he wanted. Jack and Angus Turnbull presented to me, much later, all the pre-1914 photographs used by Harts for their postcards. David Campbell contributed more of his pictures to me from time to time, as did Bruce Munro. Richard Jemmett has enlarged small snaps revealing detail, as well as adding several of his own pictures, including copies of those the Museum and Town Library allowed me to have made. A great many Waldenians living here and away have given me pictures, news cuttings and items of historical interest to whom I say again – thank you. Peter Wigley meticulously copied the photographs from the scrapbooks and to him both author and publisher are grateful.

My scrapbooks have never ceased to be of absorbing interest and they have given pleasure to many Waldenians. Therefore, when the invitation was given to me to select pictures from the collection for this book I felt I owed it to everyone to accept. I trust that all Waldenians will enjoy a peep back into the past to stir some memories and that the book will create in new-comers to Walden, that love of the old town which we have who were born in it.

H. C. Stacey

Market Place

1 The Market Square about 1790. The Market Cross (which had a sundial) on the right of the picture was a shelter for the stocks, the pillory and the whipping post. It was here that on market days usually and at the busiest hours, that sentences imposed by the magistrates at the local Sessions, took place. Stealing was almost always punished by whipping, the sentences following the form 'to be stript naked to the waste and to be tyed to the taile of a Cart and whipt till his body be bloody'. Both men and women suffered the same callous treatment. Sometimes the whipping started at the Cross, then the wretched offender was taken by the cart via a named route, often Market Hill, Church Street, High Street back to the Cross, being whipped again as in some recorded cases, outside the residence of the person sinned against – the owner of the goods stolen. These punishments for offences against the law, at a place specially provided to carry them out were intended to provide spectacles for the entertainment of the populace – in the days of 'Merrie England'.

The Market Cross was pulled down in 1818 by which time it was in a dilapidated state.

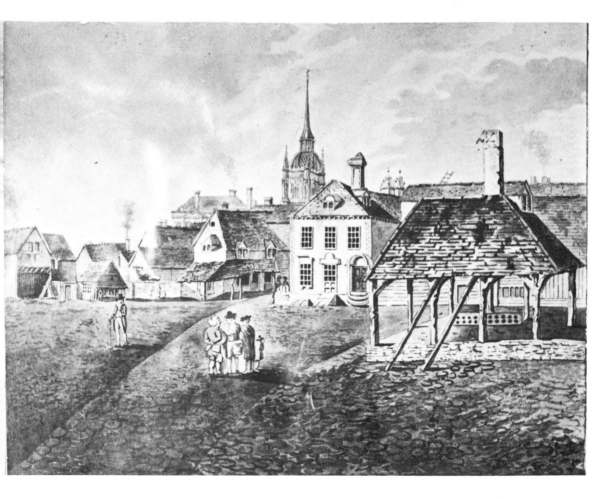

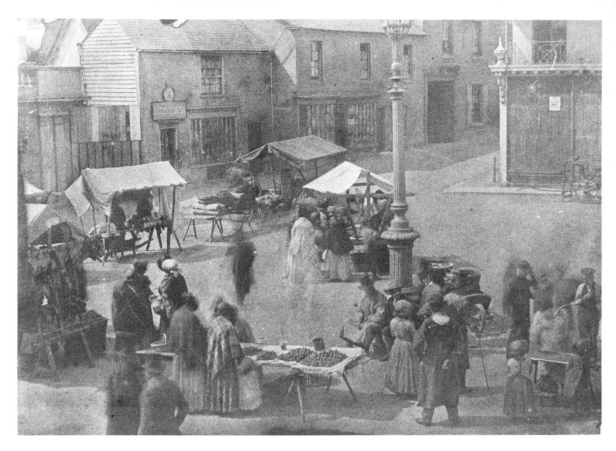

2 and 3   These 1854 pictures show the part of the Leverett property adjoining the Corn Exchange, which was to be demolished. Notice over door: *Royal Exchange Assurance Fire & Life Office*.

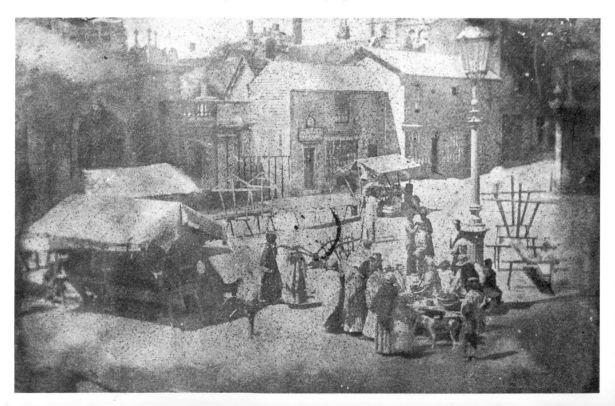

2–6 These five pictures, of considerable photographic interest, were taken in 1854 and 1855 by means of the wet-plate process introduced by Scott Archer in 1851. A long-focus lens was used (perhaps 12 inches to 15 inches) from a window above J. M. Youngman's shop (next to the Town Hall, now a wool shop), before the Court Room was built forwards from the Town Hall and over the footpath in 1879.

Taken, obviously, to show Leverett's shop (now Pennings) before and after alterations, the pictures also show the Market Square as it was in 1854/55. The stall in the NW corner is that of a rope, sack and stack-cloth maker, no doubt belonging to Henry Beans from the top of Castle Street at the entrance to Sheds Lane. Later Benjamin Beans, Gray Francis Penning had the business and for many years Mr Charles J. Langley had charge of the market stall. When H. & T. C. Godfrey bought the business they continued the stall until about 1930 when Mr Langley retired.

The street lamp in the centre of the Square was moved in 1863 to make room for the Fountain, re-erected at the top of High Street, it was removed again to make way for the War Memorial. Its new position was on the edge of the footpath where it stands today. When the Borough Council went over to electricity for street lighting, this wonderful old column was specially converted in order to preserve it. The blurred images of some of the people indicate that the picture was taken by timed exposure.

4 The shop demolished. *Note:* Two men with chimney-pot hats. One, sitting on base of lamp column, wears a smock. The simple method of making a stall with three boards on two trestles.

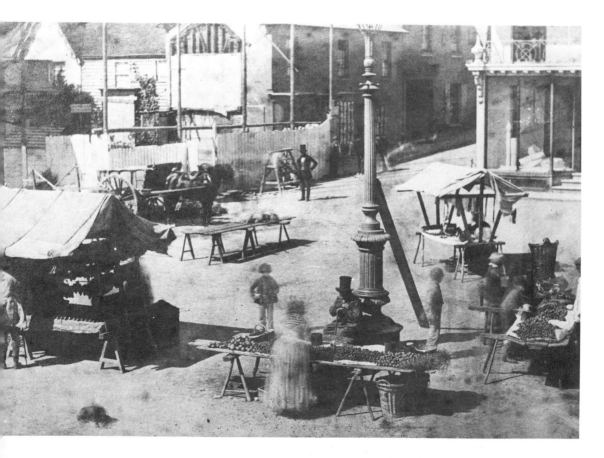

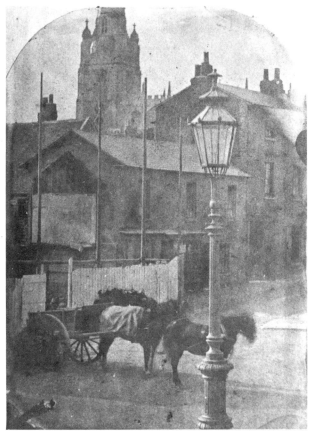

5 A wagon and two horses still clearing the site.

6 The new shop completed 1855. *Note:* goods for sale packed on ground without a stall. The 'goods' look like celery. In my boyhood days, it was usual for goods to be offered for sale without a stall. Stalls then were not supplied by the Council. The regulars had their own, the occasionals did without.

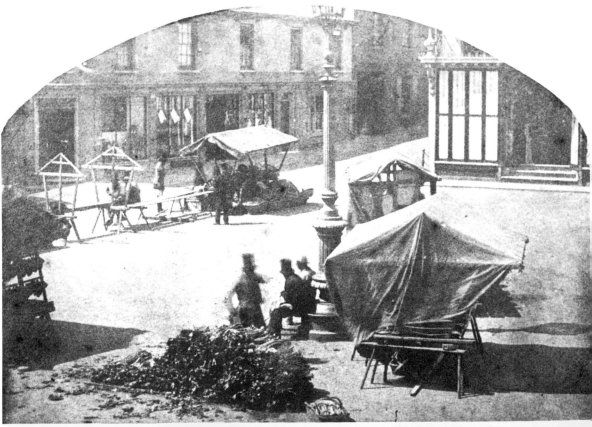

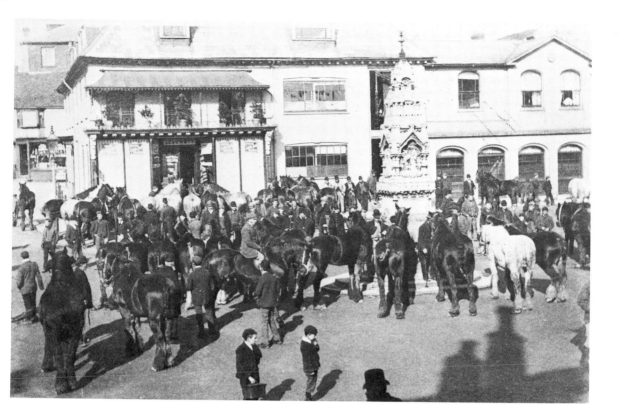

7 These Horse Fairs seem to have been started by Herbert H. Gayford, an Auctioneer and Estate Agent who lived at Hospital Farm, Newport. Just before the War in South Africa, Harold Woodward went from school to Stansted and there came into contact with Mr Gayford. They were later to be partners in business.

By 1903 Gayford and Woodward had opened a poultry market in Bishop's Stortford and in 1904 sold poultry in the Hill Street Borough Market, subject to payment of tolls. Gayford's office at this time was at 31 King Street, opposite Wabon's sweet-shop, in the property destroyed by fire *circa* 1908.

The Horse Fairs were held annually in March and September (Lady Day and Michaelmas) on the Market Place. In 1956 Mr Woodward told me that the March Fair was outstanding in the Eastern Counties, the fair comprising mostly heavy horses and vanners, George Street, King Street and the Market Place being impassable on the second of the three days. The Council collected tolls at each entrance to the town.

For 'running' the horses, dealers, according to Mr Woodward, mostly chose the narrowest streets, King Street and from Wedd's Coach Showroom in George Street to Guy's papershop in Cross Street, the latter being the most popular.

Among the dealers most respected for their integrity were Mr Duke of Chishill, Mr Duke of Trumpington and Mr Emson of Bumpstead. The Dukes were always located at *The White Horse*, Mr Emson in front of Barclays Bank. Buyers from many of the great haulage firms of London amd most of the Railway Companies were in attendance with several from the Midlands, Birmingham, Rugby, etc. For some years Mr Woodward conducted the auctions at these March Fairs 'when the confidence built up over many years between men of standing amongst the breeders and representatives of the haulage companies, was so sound that the best animals found a direct sale'.

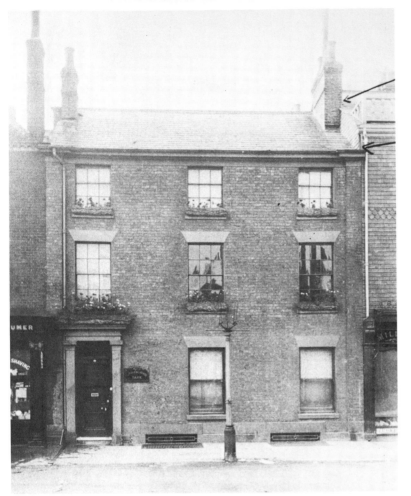

8 No 3 Market Place. The London & County Bank, now National Westminster Bank.

9 This picture, I would guess, was taken in the early 1920s before the Market Place came to be an official parking place. The charabanc was probably on an excursion trip, parking while the passengers visited the *Rose and Crown*. The charabanc would appear to have solid rubber tyres. The driver is inspecting his engine.

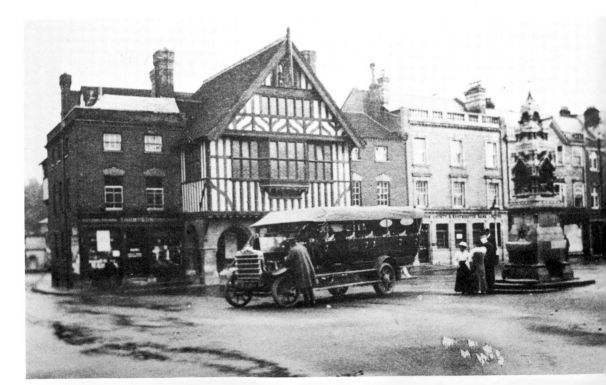

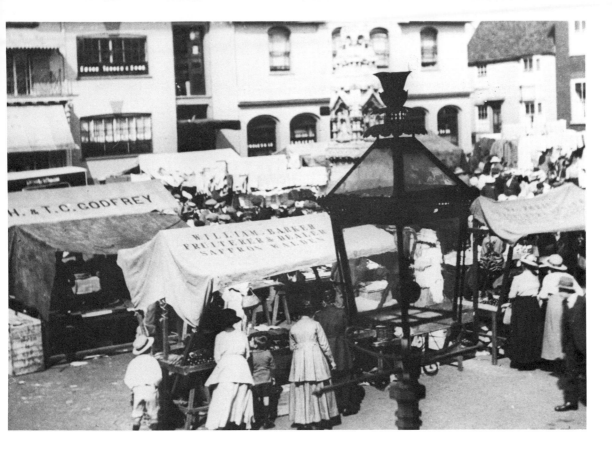

10 Market Day *circa* 1920. William (*Soldier*) Barker's stall occcupied the same corner pitch on the Square for many years. Bill Parish's was next to it.

Godfrey's stall always occupied the NW corner site. It was the traditional pitch for the town's rope and sack makers, stack-covers, etc, back to the times of Henry Beans, Benjamin Beans and Gray Francis Penning carried on at the bottom of Sheds Lane. Before the 1914–18 War, George Lee of Thaxted was a 'regular', with his large sweet stall on the east side of the Square, facing the Bank. All Lee's sweets were made at Thaxted. It was at this stall we spent our Saturday penny.

Market Hill

11 1925. No 17, at the corner of Church Street (top right), was occupied by Mrs Arnold who came from Elmdon with her two daughters, to open the Cromwell Tea Rooms. At No 14 opposite, Mr Couper had followed Mr Goodfellow with a toyshop, etc.

The *Green Dragon* (now Trustees Savings Bank), was at this time still a licensed inn. When the magistrates refused to renew the licence, the sign was transferred to Sewards End. The vacated inn was then taken over by Teddy Worley, who moved there from Cates Corner where he had his saddler's business.

The shop (No 13) outside which the car stands, was the Gibsons' 'Saffron Walden and North-Essex Bank', opened in 1824. It remained there until 1874, when it moved to new premises in the Market Place, known then as 'Gibson, Tuke & Gibson Bank. The vacated property in Market Hill became the post office where it stayed until 1888 when it moved to King Street (now W. H. Smith & Son).

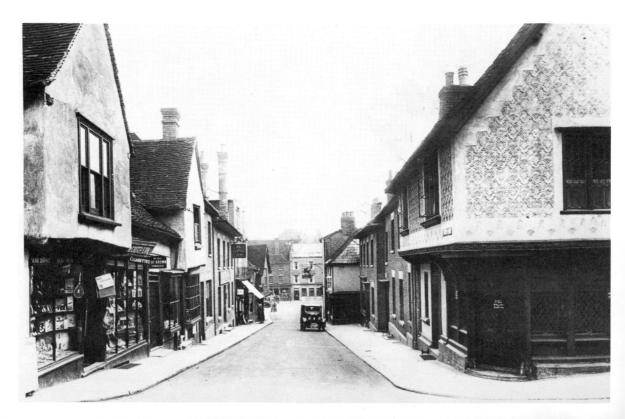

Mercers Row

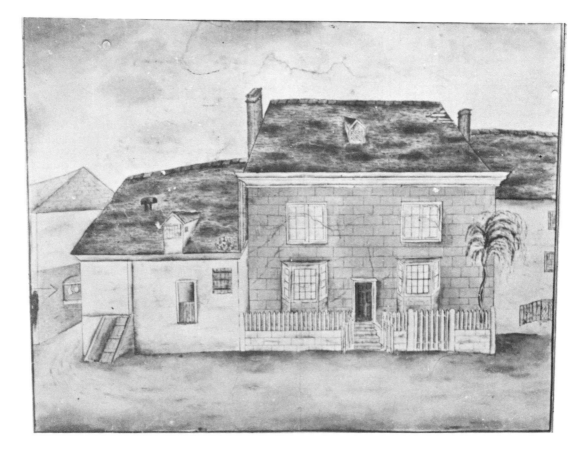

12   This is a photo-copy of a watercolour picture I found in the Museum Library (now in the Town Library) on which was recorded that the original was in the possession of Charles Hagger, Antiques Dealer. The house is the one which stood at the eastern end of Mercers Row, next *The Dolphin* inn until it was acquired by the Corporation in 1840 to provide a lock-up house more suitable than the one in use at that time. The lane behind the Town Hall (the one built in 1761 not the present one built 1879) was blocked up by Court Order. *The Dolphin* moved to Gold Street to the property now No 6 opposite the Steam Laundry offices. The inn sign can still be seen in the plaster-work of the house. The road on the left is Butcher Row and the property on the right *The Dolphin.*

King Street

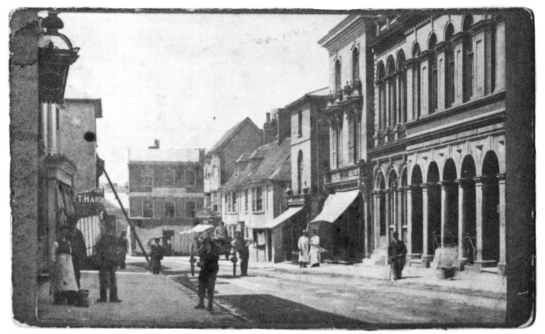

13   This picture was taken before the re-building of the area between Harts and Lime Tree Passage in 1888.
It also shows the Literary and Scientific Institution (now Town Library) before the alteration of the frontage and the conversion into a shop (now A. James Ltd) of a semi-private house.

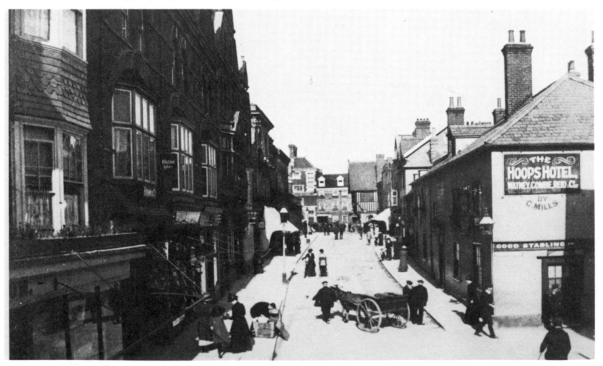

14   The photograph was taken from over Walter Robson's furniture shop, *circa* 1912. The large company of men on the Market Square suggests to me that a Horse Fair was being held.

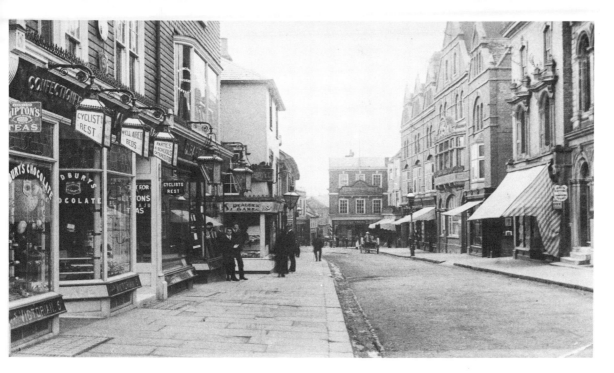

15 *Circa* 1910. F. J. Taylor's *Victorian Cafe* on the left, David Barton Gent's Outfitters next (photographer's son, Mansell Jnr, with Bert Pateman by window). On the opposite side of the road, the house next the library was in the occupation, not of the librarian, but of Mr G. D. Dobson, the hairdresser, who, about this time, moved to the premises No 17–19 King Street, at the corner of Cross Street and which still bears his name. C. E. Spurge had the draper's next door. *Note:* the milk cart outside Stead and Simpson's shop.

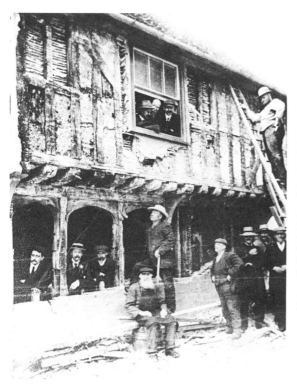

16 There is little doubt that what we know today as Nos 17, 19 and 21 King Street, was one 'hall house', probably the home of a wealthy resident.

In 1906 Walter Robson owned Nos 17 and 19 and decided to strip off the plaster and expose the oak timbers. He engaged Ben Dix, Builder of 10 High Street to do the work.

Timothy Hunt of Newport, J. W. Burningham and Guy Maynard are at the top window, Jim Surrey on the ladder; David Gillett sits on the plank; Ben Dix stands behind him; Chas Mills of *Hoops* stands at the foot of the ladder. Ben Newell of Newport is the man first on left and I believe John Hills (Castle Street) and Jim Pateman (Butcher) are sixth and seventh from left.

After the alterations were completed, George Daniel Dobson, who had had his hairdresser's business at No 4 King Street (later the librarian's house) became the tenant of Nos 17 (shop) and 19 (house). Previously Mr T. Scales (late Peter Wedd), saddler and harness maker, had occupied the property.

Mr Scales moved to Market Passage (now the Coffee House behind Hardwicks) and later to the shop next the *White Horse*.

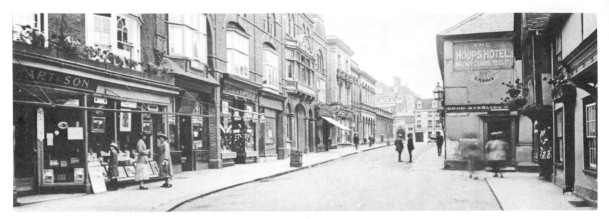

17 *Circa* 1920. Shows Harts, still with the familiar flowers above the shop front. The next shop, Brown & Co, sold cycles and did repairs; Stead & Simpson; Empire Meat Co; Cleales; Mrs E. Warren, high-class dress shop; Lime Tree Passage leading to the solicitors' office of Ackland, Son & Baily and office of Saffron Walden Building Society; C. E. Spurge.

In the early days of World War I plans were laid in case the country was invaded. To secure that the population should evacuate in the same direction, white arrows were painted on the walls of properties indicating the direction we should all go. One such arrow can be seen on the wall of *The Hoops* pointing down Cross Street.

By this time Mr Dobson the hairdresser had moved down the street and librarian A. E. Gower was residing in No 4.

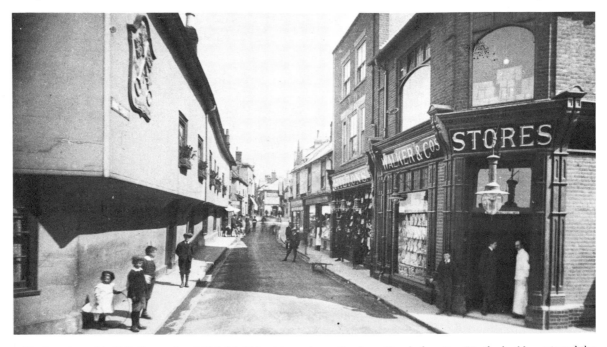

18 Junction with High Street *circa* 1912–14. This picture shows the *Cross Keys* before Ben Dix the builder stripped the plaster and exposed the timbers. If any reader can tell me the exact date of this photograph I would appreciate the information

In 1709 the *Cross Keys* was called the *Bull's Head*, but sixty years later the property was described in the title deeds as a 'Baking Office'. By 1778, however, the house had come back into its own, taking the sign *Cross Keys*. In recent years a claim has been made that the house was reputed to have carried the sign of *The Whalebone*, but the title deeds do not confirm this.

Walkers Stores was built and opened in about 1907 on the site of Beard & Son, Drapers. The Beard's private house was No 30 (now Eastern Electric).

Hiltons (Bootmakers), No 37, King Street, next to Walkers, was opened in about 1908 with Mr W. C. de Barr as manager. Arthur Titchmarsh had a provisions and wine store at No 35 and Arthur James, watchmaker and jeweller, was at No 33. No 31 (Home & Colonial Stores) was set back 5–6 feet. F. R. Furlong (gunsmith) had his shop and private house between the *Cross Keys* yard and J. Dominick (hardware and ironmongery).

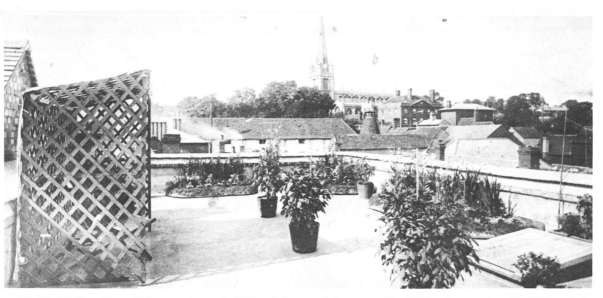

19 No 37 King Street. Taken on the roof of Hilton's boot and shoe shop, No 37 King Street, when Mr Walter C. de Barr was manager and lived over the shop. High Street lies along the left of the picture and King Street across the centre. The long plastered building with the kiln at the east end was Barnards Yard. The tall house next to the kiln was *Dorset House*. The picture was taken about 1913.

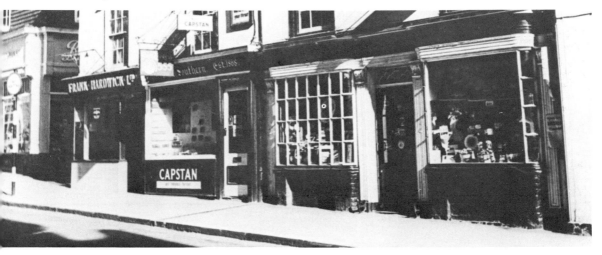

20 Nos 7–11, *circa* 1950. At this time No 7 was Boots the chemists, No 9 the long-established fishmongers Frank Hardwick and No 11 was owned by Silvester Southern.

From as early as 1887 to about 1914, Mrs Eliza Smith and her four daughters lived at No 13, the two front rooms, left and right of the centre door, being used for business purposes. In one Miss Julia ran a hairdressing business and in the other Miss Kate had an employment agency. She also sold toys and cutlery but discontinued from doing so during the 1914–18 War. Edith married and left Walden. Charlotte worked for David Barton in his Ladies' Dress Shop next to the Westminster Bank and by 1914 she had set up her own well-patronised business as a dressmaker and costumier at 5 Market Row.

The room on the right was let to Mr S. A. Chilton who opened up as a tobacconist and confectioner. After World War II Mr Southern's son, Bill, took over Chilton's business and also Miss Smith's room on the left.

The plate-glass window on the right, put in by Mr Chilton, had come under criticism for spoiling the appearance of this old property, and Bill himself did not like the alteration. When carrying out internal improvements he instructed his architect to install a new window to match the one on the left

When paint was scraped from one of the curved ends of the left-hand window the wood was found to be of mahogany, so the frame of the right-hand window was made of the same wood and fitted. The intention was to strip all the paint off the left-hand window, treating it to match the new right-hand one. However, the front section between the curved ends was found to be of ordinary deal, and so both windows had to be painted white.

Thanks to David Campbell's picture this little-known story serves to illustrate the commendable action of a King Street trader who, having accepted that the frontage appearance of this old property had been spoiled, voluntarily rectified it.

21 Hart's Yard 1904. Gateway between Hepworths and Chew and Osborne, as it was in 1904. The building at the top of the yard was Hart's printing office with Hart's garden to the right of it.

Over the top of the gateway is a room to which there appears to be no access except by a ladder from the yard below.

Before Hepworths came to the town, the shop was the furniture and hardware department of Walter Robson who had his drapery, millinery, footwear department, on the other side of King Street. Robsons used the premises in Church Street (now the Masonic Hall) as a furniture depository and during the 1914–18 War, the YMCA, in High Street, for the same purpose.

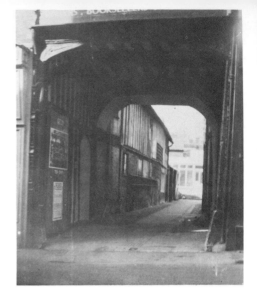

22 Looking up Hart's Yard. J. Dominick's on the left and Walter Robson's furniture shop on the right, the Yard between led to W. E. Hart's garden at the rear of No 18. The shed at the end of the Yard was Hart's printing works, later to be much improved and extended.

The building on the left, halfway up the Yard, was the *Tailor's Arms*, destroyed by fire in November 1930, I believe. It was not a licensed inn in my time.

The gateway entrance to the Yard is a 'listed' property described as originally forming part of 'a late 15th-century house built on a half H-shaped plan with wings extending north on either side of a wagon way which still remains'.

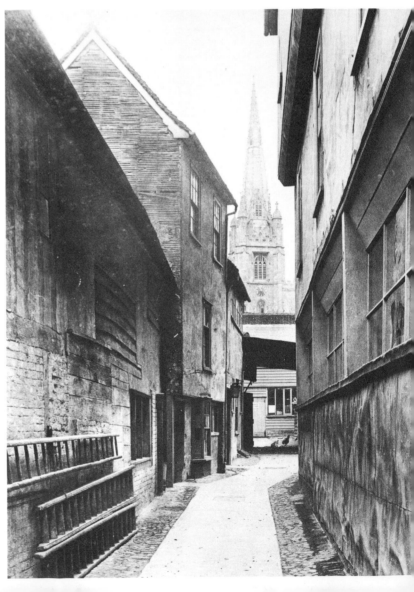

George Street

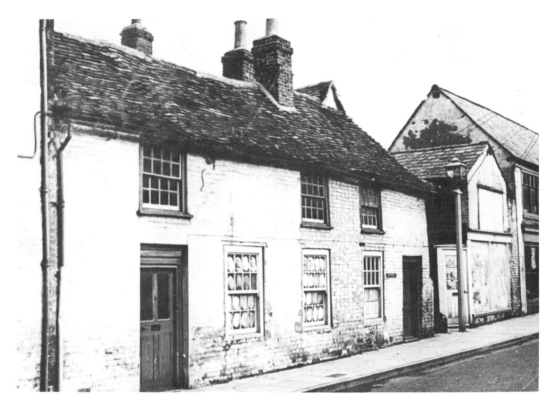

23 The first house was next to A. V. Britton's slaughterhouse. The second house was occupied by Mrs Emily Hagger and her daughter Agnes when they had the former Wedd Coachbuilder's showroom seen at the end, as their antiques shop. Charles Hagger moved here from 41–43 Castle Street. The Haggers later moved from George Street to 57 High Street.

Gold Street

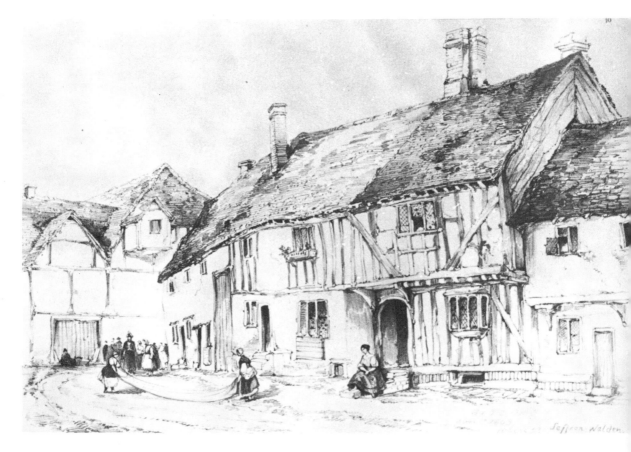

24   T. C. Dibdin's drawing of the southern end of Gold Street made in 1843, showing the women with their silk crêpe, a home-industry in the town at this time. The drawing can be compared with the post-war photograph (plate 111).

No 40 (John Bacon's fish shop) can, I think, be identified up to the first break in the roof. Nos 42, 44 and 46 would appear to be new. Nos 48 and 50 on the bend, and perhaps the cottages round the corner (Nos 52–58) may perhaps have escaped reconstruction.

Before Bacon took over No 40 and altered the front, Walter J. Housden (Plumber, Painter and Decorator) lived there and before him Alfred Evenett had a fish, fruit and vegetable shop there.

25 *Circa* 1900. Showing 'Wm. Day & Co., Castle Brewery' notice on building on which site the present Steam Laundry was built.

A woman looks to be buying something from the man in the cart. The woman on the pavement is probably going to do the same. Perhaps it was the man who, in my time, used to drive his cart round the town with a load of peas, shouting 'Peas, fourpence a peck', varying the cry with 'Pea-pods' or 'Pods' and of course, the price.

It will be noted that the property in George Street looking up Gold Street was a private house. In my boyhood days, Stan (*Marley*) Day's mother had a little sweet-shop on the curve of the building. To the right of it was Wm Lovell's eating-place, at 2–4 Cross Street. Mr Lovell played the double bass in the Town Band and his daughter gave me my first piano lessons when the family lived at 3 Abbey Lane.

As a boy, I looked forward to Friday tea-times during the winter months because that was the day Lovell's cooked-meat shop sold 'faggots'. I used to take a pudding basin and tea towel in a basket and trot down to Cross Street about 5 o'clock, put my basin on the counter and wait until the lady came out with one or more piping hot faggots in it, to be covered with the cloth and taken home to Castle Street in double quick time. At that age I couldn't have told you what a 'faggot' was and I can't now. I suppose it was a kind of rissole covered with gravy. Be that as it may, it was a tasty morsel and something I looked forward to – like I did Sillett's hot 'puffs' for breakfast! They were indigestible, but lovely grub.

Addy Nunn Myhill's corn and seeds and coal business was on the left-hand side.

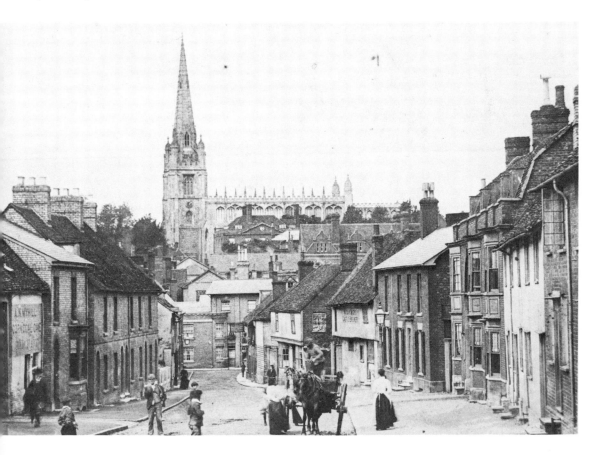

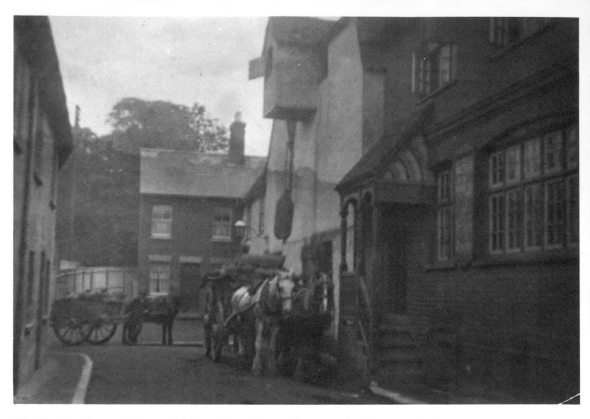

26 The *Sun*. Wagons delivering barley at the malting in that part of Gold Street which was previously called *Powell's Corner*. There were other maltings in Gold Street, some pulled down, others to find new uses.

Early in World War II, these disused maltings were taken over by J. Sainsbury, who evacuated from one of their London grocery and provision warehouses into the country. A fire on 12 July 1941, destroyed the part of the malting shown in this picture.

When the site was cleared after the fire, the area between the *Sun* and No 53 was made into a loading and unloading area for the warehouse behind. This loading bay can be seen in plate number 111.

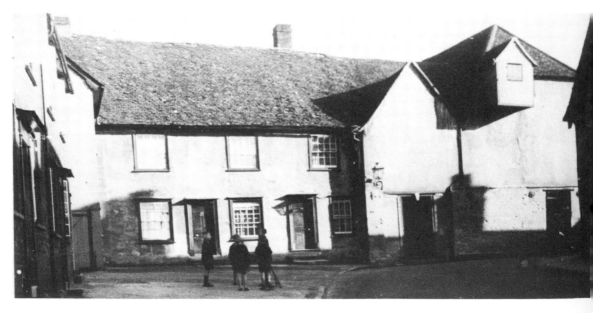

27 The south end of the street. The house in the corner occupied by Bill Dennis is No 51 and the house in the picture is No 53. The malting lying between No 53 and the *Sun Inn*, was destroyed by fire in the early part of the 1939–45 War.

Museum Street

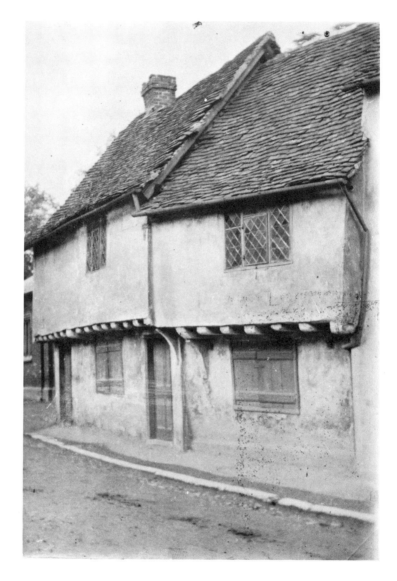

28 Two cottages which would have been Nos 11 and 13 Museum Street were demolished 1894, the site providing a playground for the Museum Street Infants' School which can just be seen at the back of the picture. There is a curve in the road here which makes the picture deceptive.

The present No 9 called *Cobbler's Cottage* is misnamed because Mr A. E. Wright, the cobbler and secretary of the Shepherds Club, lived at No 7.

Castle Street

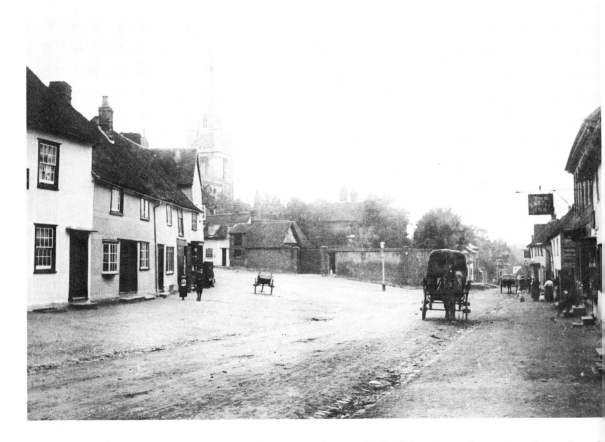

29 Junction with Museum Street *circa* 1912. This is a view showing the *Castle Inn* sign –today a private house. It used to be a licensed doss-house or common lodging house where the police would direct tramps to go, if they would not go into the Workhouse.

Mrs Harriett Reader had the shop next the *Castle Inn* before she moved higher up the street. Charlie Farnham succeeded her.

When the Market Cross in the Market Square was demolished in 1818, the stocks were moved to about where the street lamp is in the picture. From there they went to the Castle.

In one of the Museum Street cottages – No 4 – I remember E. H. Kenny lived. He made medicines for cattle and poultry.

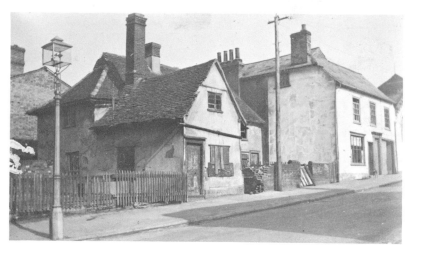

30   The fenced off entrance to School Row; No 93 Castle Street; Nos 95 and 97 standing back between Nos 93 and 99.
    No 99 was the grocery shop of Mr Charles Adams, before it was taken over by the Co-operative Society. Mr Adams's *Snowflake Laundry* (1907–68) adjoined No 99 and is seen only at the edge of the picture. Originally the site of *The Black Horse*, the Salvation Army established their headquarters in the building which became the laundry. William Barker, a greengrocer of 63 Castle Street and a regular stall-holder on the market, was a member of the Salvation Army and everyone knew him as *Soldier* Barker.

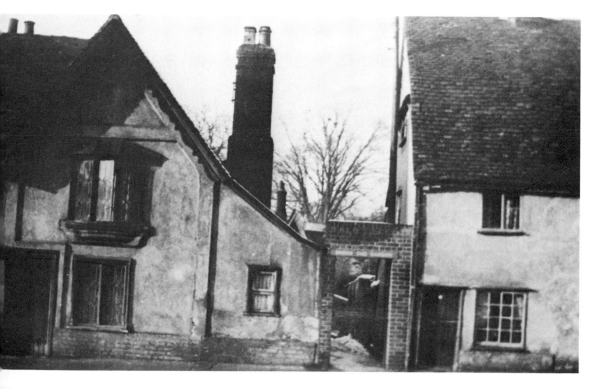

31   Nos 19 and 23 Castle Street with entrance to Fry's Gardens and No 21. Nos 23 and 25 were converted into one house in 1966.

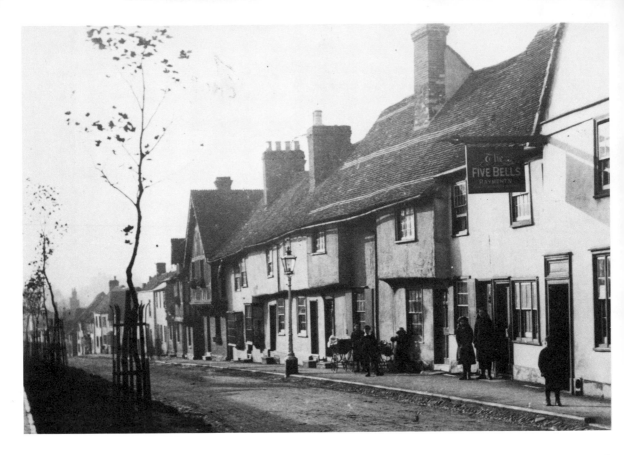

32 *Five Bells* westwards *circa* 1920. Richard (*Dick*) Goddard left the *Five Bells* in 1920 to be succeeded by Mrs Smith. Judy Smith and her sister stand outside the Bottle and Jug entrance. *Note:* The gutters of cobblestones; roads not yet tarmacadam treated. The fairly recently planted trees. The boat-shaped high-wheeeled prams. The shoe-scraper by the *Five Bells* main door.

Church Street

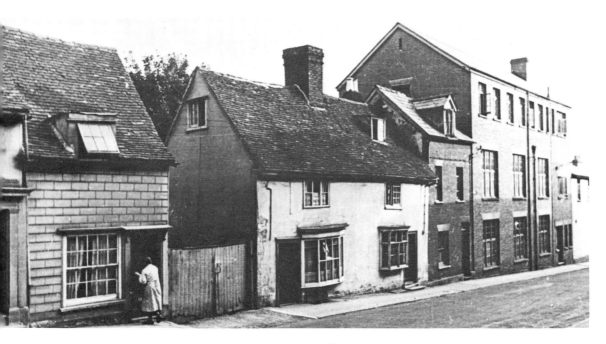

33 Nos 11, 9, 7, 5, 3, and Cambridge House. No 3 formed part of Miss Gowlett's School but when the school finished it became a privately let cottage. Nos 5 and 7 were demolished September 1956 to February 1957. George Moore lived at No 5 when he was a boy. No 9 was a small house used in my boyhood days by the mail van driver.

Eventually Nos 9 and 11 came to be occupied as one house, the door of No 9 has in fact been blocked up.

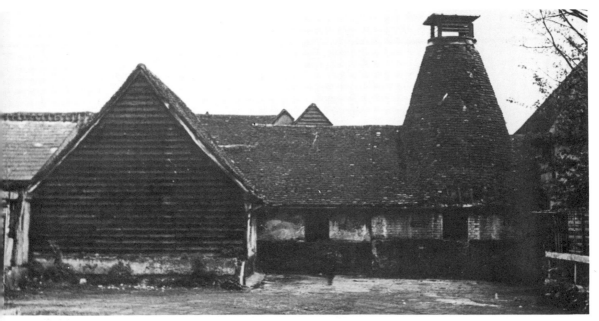

34 The old Malting in Barnard's yard, High Street, as seen through the open site of the demolished Nos 5 and 7 Church Street.

Church Path

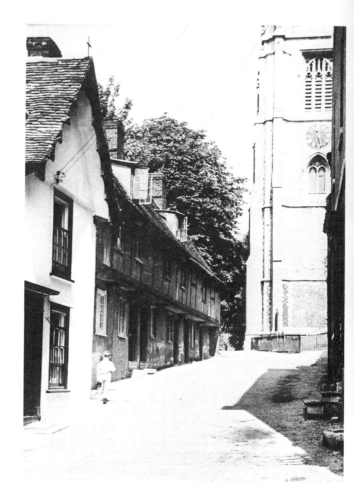

35 1939 before conversion in 1958. This picture shows the iron railings round the church burial grounds, removed in the early days of the 1939–45 War.

It is held by church historians that the larger part of the churchyard was always on the south side of the church so that the church's shadow should not fall on the graves.

In the late 1920s a trench was dug 2 to 3 feet from the wall of Dorset House to take an electricity cable to the church, I believe. I remember seeing many human bones disturbed by the workmen digging at even shallow depths. As far down Church Path as the turning into Church Street, almost at the corner of Dorset House, a small skeleton was found amd among my souvenirs I still have the vertebra bone I picked out of the trench. From this evidence it seems a fair assumption that the churchyard originally extended southwards at least to the present Church Street. It should be remembered that a Walden Church existed in 1136 because it was one of the 19 churches assigned by Geoffrey de Mandeville when he founded a monastery in Walden and one can go back even earlier – to 1066 when William the Conqueror granted the Church property in Walden to one of his supporters, Geoffrey de Mandeville, grandfather of the founder of Walden Abbey.

In medieval days, the churchyard or 'God's Acre' (the customary area) was used on Feast Days for dancing and games and it was the venue for other activities.

The rear yard of the cottages was through a passage to the left of the boy in the picture. The rooms at the back were at a lower level than those in the front

The cottage at the left hand-corner is now occupied by the publishers of this book.

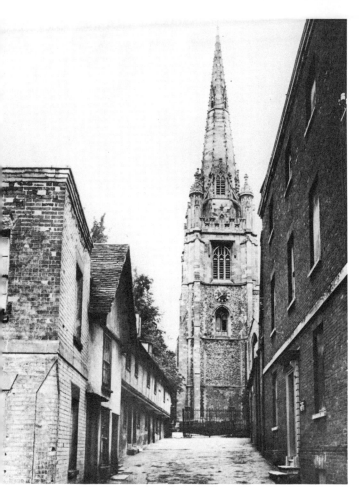

36 Taken in the 1920s after the building at the far end of Dorset House had been converted into a billiards room with windows opening into Church Path. The end entrance on right at the Church Street corner was the part occupied by the Territorials. The heavy iron gates into the churchyard, with smaller gates on each side, were removed during the 1939–45 War to help make munitions.

37 Taken in 1957 from the churchyard looking down east side of Dorset House. Before the 1939–45 War, the Territorials had their headquarters in the corner of Dorset House with entrance at the far end.

The regular army sergeant in charge (Sgt Miller, after Sgt Worrell, I think) lived at the top of their quarters. The Comrades Club first, then the Area Guardians Committee (Percy H. Wright, Clerk) Relieving Officer and Registrar of Births, etc, (Stanley Read), occupied the other part of Dorset House, with access from the main front door in Church Street

The one-storey building at the church end with access through a passage in the front of the car, was converted into a billiards room.

Joseph Bell, who died 30 December 1911, was, I believe, the last person to occupy the house as a private resident.

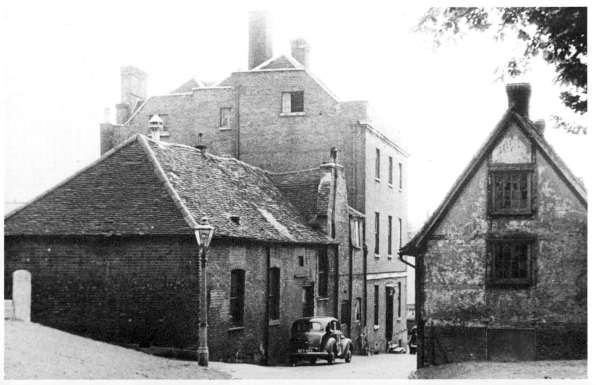

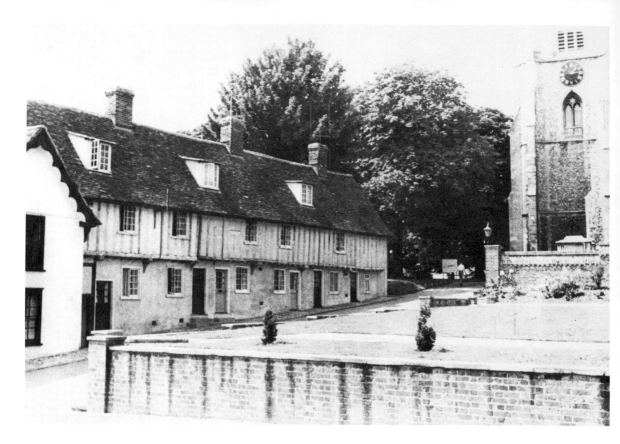

38 After the 1958 conversion. No 1 is the house at the Church Street corner. The original 6 cottages were converted into three, each having two doors, being Nos 2, 3 and 4.

The opening at the church end of No 1 is a passage leading to the rear yard of the three dwellings.

High Street

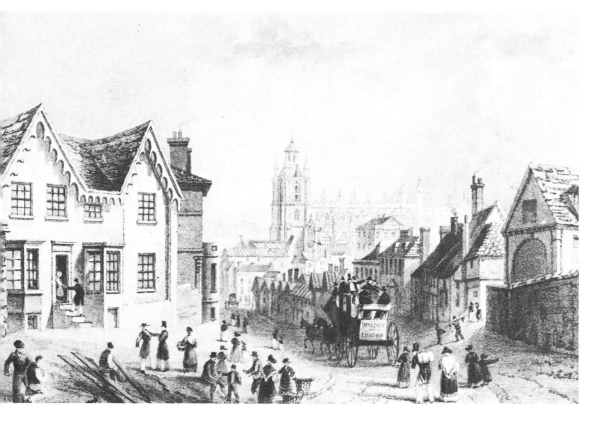

39 Cuckingstool End Street, *circa* 1820. Early last century, the Vestry, to provide employment, used to set men 'on the roads' for wages instead of giving them poor relief for doing nothing in return. In 1807/08 Windmill Hill was much improved. In 1826 it was decided to lower and improve the London Road (as Newport Road was then called) 'near Burntwoman's Closes'. There was then a hard road from the Claypits in Debden Road following what today we call Seven Devils' Lane (the hedges on each side of the road at the east end of this public footpath have survived) crossing the London highway (now the Newport Road 'cutting') over Sedcop Hill to Audley End hamlet. The Burntwoman's Closes were on both sides of the London Road at the cross-over of the Claypits Road.

Inspection of both sides of Newport Road from its junction with Borough Lane to the top of Sparrows End Hill will reveal many ups and downs in the contours. The banks, some below, some above road level, are evidence for the person with time to stand and stare, of the pronounced switchback nature of the original road. In May 1827, there was so much unemployment that the Vestry decided on further improvements by lowering the hill between the 'Porthbridge' at the bottom of Gallows Hill (the Fulfen or Beechy Ride) to the borough boundary at the top of Sparrows End Hill. Newport Parish Council were invited to co-operate in the undertaking by lowering such part of the road as lay in that parish. They did not respond nor, apparently, did they do so when they were approached again in June 1829 when the whole new Gallows Hill Road was lined with stones 6 inches thick, 18 feet wide.

Apart from providing work to save the handing out of poor relief, the Vestry hoped the improvements would encourage the mail coaches from Cambridge to London to pass through Walden. In that, however, they failed, for the coaches preferred the level main road from Littlebury to Newport.

With this dip into the history of Newport Road, readers can now ponder on the precarious up hill, down dale, route of the London–Walden stage coach shown in the picture, especialy in wintertime. We can also marvel at the engineering feat performed in the pick and shovel, horse and cart days.

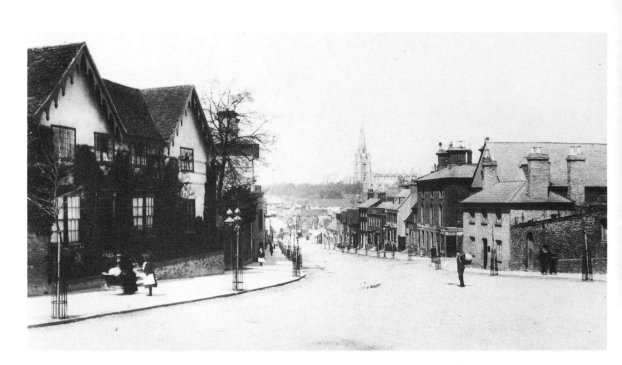

40 *Circa* 1905. The trees were planted in March 1902 and it is from their appearance that I date this picture.

The Gables, complete with iron railings, shows the front well covered with the lovely wisteria I remember. In the wall at the left edge of the picture there used to be a letter-box.

The sunblind at the bottom of High Street is outside the Co-op which was built and opened for business 16 March 1905.

No 82, at the corner of Gold Street (formerly Powell's Corner) would seem to have been a shop at this time. A private house originally, old photographs show sometimes a bricked-up rounded corner, sometimes a shop door. It has changed with its occupation, obviously depending on whether the front room was to be used for business purposes or as a sitting-room.

The Walden Cinema was not built until 1912.

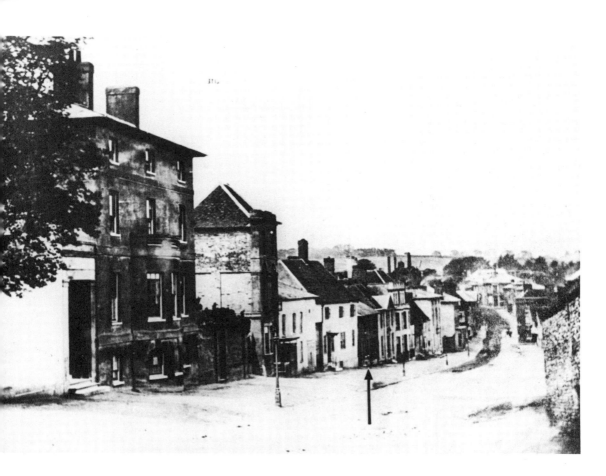

41 Cuckingstool End Street (name changed to High Street about 1814). The original part of *Hill House* was built in 1821 by Henry Archer. George Stacey Gibson married Elizabeth Tuke in 1845, bought the house and at some stage enlarged it extensively and called it Hill House.

I would think G. S. G. added the entrance door, conservatory, etc, on the south side before 1862 the reputed date of this picture and afterwards extended on the north end.

The original house had two rows of three upper windows which were not matched by the upper windows in the extension.

Trees in the High Street were not planted until 1902. The one in the picture was one growing in the Hill House Garden and overhanging the wall.

The arrow points to the three cottages, the site of the 1879 Friends' Meeting House.

42 Top of the High Street looking west along London Road *circa* 1900. This picture was given to me by Arthur W. Parker whose family lived in South Road. The young lady on the bicycle is Arthur's sister and the picture was taken about 6 am.

The alley-way east of the shop leads through to Albert Place (later to be called *Ingleside Place*) consisting of 16 cottages which were demolished under the Council's slum clearance Order made just before the 1939–45 War, and the tenants rehoused in Little Walden Road.

The four terraced houses (Nos 88, 89, 90 and 92) are shown in the picture as plastered. Not long after, they were brick-faced.

The Churchwardens and Vestry, in 1734, acquired for a Workhouse, property described as 'commonly called or known by the name or sign of the *White Hart* formerly two messuages . . . in or near a street called Cuckingstool End Street between the messuage of . . . Stacey on the east and the messuage of Henry Dalliston on the west fronting north on Cuckingstool End Street and on the south on ground called Lime Kiln Yard'.

This row which, after refacing, was called *Ingleside Terrace*, was the Workhouse but the above *White Hart* was not the inn where Samuel Pepys stayed when he visited Audley End on 27 February 1659. At that time the *White Hart*, according to manorial records, stood on the site of Cambridge House at the corner of Church Street/High Street.

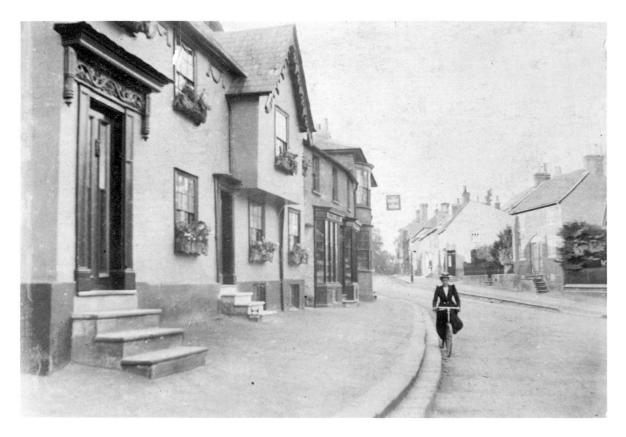

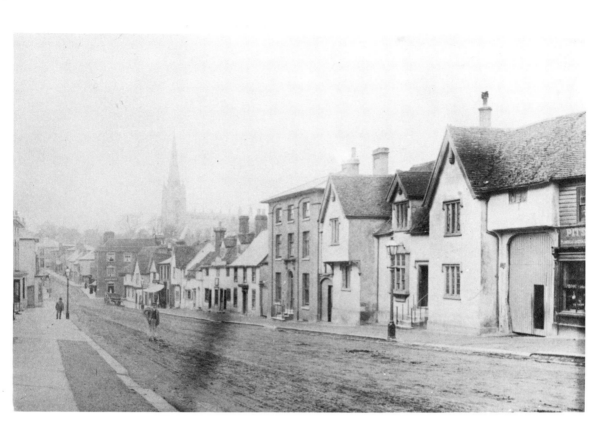

43 Before the trees were planted in 1902 and when W. H. Day, Wood Turner and Cabinet Maker was there before Choppens at No 58, *circa* 1895.

No 66 Fred Pitstow, Painter and Decorator, Plumber; 64 John Hughes, Coachbuilder; 62 E. W. Trew, Draper, etc (Tally-man); 60 Priscilla Anne Barrett, 58 W. H. Day (who had gone by 1900 by which year J. A. Choppen had not arrived; 56 Henry Thos Gatward, Watchmaker; 54 James Costin; 52 Frank Clayden (but not until 1910).

Note: that at the time of this picture, No 64 had not been brick-faced. There was a big fire there about 1912 (plate 48) so perhaps the brick-facing formed part of the repair work (see plate 47).

44 From George Street looking southwards *circa* 1910. The notice boards in front of the *Greyhound* on the left belong to Mr C. W. Charter, Bill Poster.

The Mace Bearer and Town Crier usually filled up his time bill-posting and it was in his interests to rent hoardings or get permission to stick his bills on properties at vantage points in town and surrounding villages. In the 1930s these hoardings had rental values and were accordingly rated.

The lady with the large hat and bicycle is, I believe, the wife of Walter Francis who had his photographer's business next to the Co-op (now De Barr's).

The small child in the entrance to the *Greyhound* is probably Muriel, the daughter of the licensee, Mr T. J. Pledger. The boy, standing with the girl, is the son of H. Mansell, the photographer.

The posters advertise a Woodward and Priday furniture sale at Newport; the same firm's horses sale on the 12 October; and Lord John Sangers' Circus.

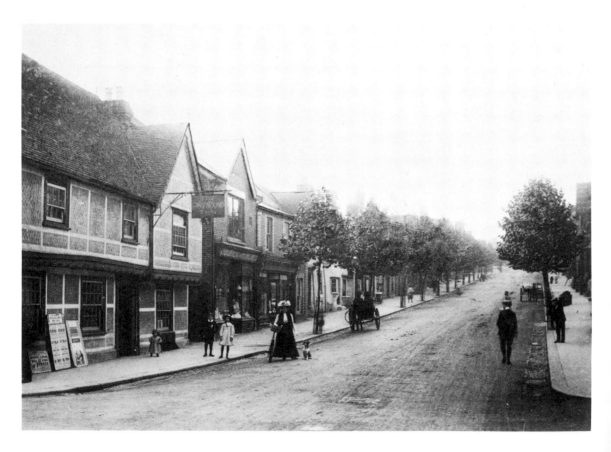

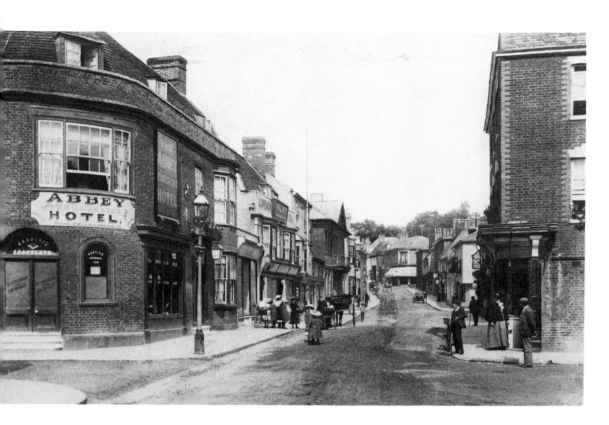

45 Before the corner of the *Cross Keys* was stripped of its plaster and the timbers exposed, about 1910.

A. G. Edward was the proprietor of the *Abbey Temperance Hotel*. He was followed by P. F. Scotney.

The door on the left of the picture used to be the entrance to the room where one could buy a coffee and sandwich, but later access was by the main High Street door.

The small door a little further down Abbey Lane led upstairs to a long room where, in childhood days, there used to be held 6½d bazaars once or twice a year. The vendor was not local but brought his goods of china, crockery, kitchen requisites, brushes, etc, nothing over 6½d – a forerunner of the Woolworth method of trade 'Nothing over sixpence in the store'. The thing I remember most is the bran-tub and the delight of diving one's hand in the bran to find some trifling toy.

'Nicholls' was in the shop next to the *Abbey Hotel*, soon after to be Walbro's cycle shop. Mr Ernest Street stands in the doorway of his draper's shop.

The door into Willett's butcher's shop is, in this picture, on the corner. Older pictures show the doorway further to the right in George Street.

The photographer has painted out on his plate the man on a bicycle with a front carrier and a basket in it. Note the blur. Note also, the very small motor vehicle with a boy standing beside it, outside Joe Wright's.

46 *Circa* 1920. Originally, High Street extended from King Street corner to Castle Street junction. From King Street to George Street was 'Middle Ward' and from George Street to Debden Road 'Cuckingstool End Street'.

The house on the left belonged to Dr J. P. Atkinson Snr, who died 1917. The Post Office bought the property, converted into a post office and moved into it from King Street soon after the war ended. Mr Whalley of Bishop's Stortford bought the King Street post office and it is his sign-board 'To Ford Service Depot Phone 62' which hangs on Walkers Stores.

A 1620 Manorial Rental includes the *Swan Inn* as standing on the site of the post office.

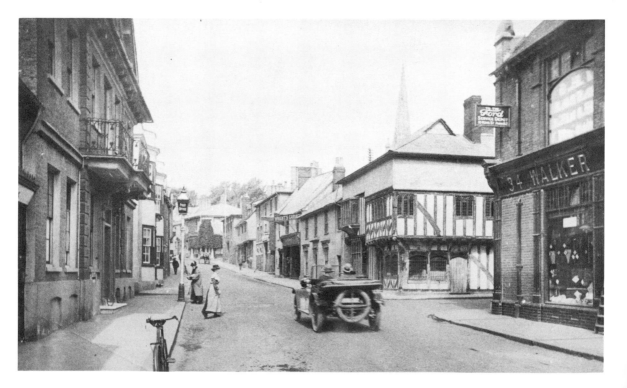

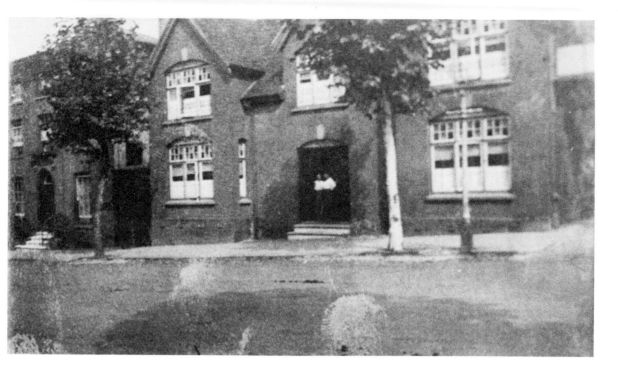

47 Nos 62 and 64 High Street. After Mr E. W. Trew, a Draper (Tally-man) moved from No 62 to 86 High Street, Mrs Fred Vert (a widow) converted No 62 into a boarding house. It was well patronised for it met a need for that kind of accommodation. Later, Miss Muriel Pledger had it to maintain its reputation. Today, Frank Bacon has his wet fish and greengrocery shop there.

Before No 64 was converted into a motor showroom for Walden Motors Ltd, it was the private house of Mr Frank Bailey who had his garage and motor repairs shop and yard at the back. There was a little shop on the right-hand side of the yard entrance where motor accessories could be obtained and petrol from an overhead feed.

In the early 1920s Mr E. A. Kett, electrician, had this shop and Ted Peasgood and Monty Watson were his young assistants. 'Wireless' was coming into the picture. Mr Kett was experimenting in the workshop overhead with these new-fangled cat whiskers, reaching the stage eventually when he could relay this remarkable invention. He built a loudspeaker into one of the windows above the shop and when the 'wireless' gave out the news, he tuned in and boosted the sound so that it could be heard on the other side of High Street. Crowds of people gathered to hear it and it undoubtedly boosted the sale of cat-whisker sets. Ted Peasgood earned a reputation for himself as a 'wireless man' – radio engineer in today's terms. Monty Watson emigrated, I think, to Canada.

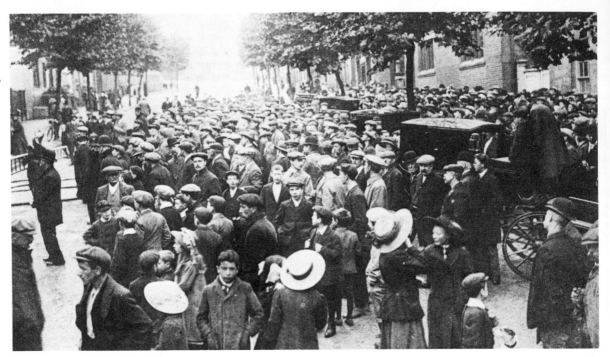

48 Fire at Hughes' Coachbuilders, behind No 64, now Walden Motors, before 1914. There are three carriages in the crowd gathered to watch the fire. It was rather a disastrous one. I can recognise in the crowd Police Sergeant Brown, Walter Pettitt, 'Mother' Cox, Jim Dennis, Coote and Shelley.

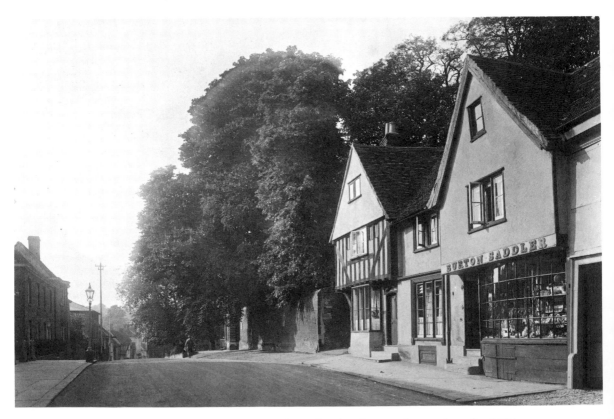

49 Nos 4 and 6 High Street. The electricity poles indicate that the photograph was taken after 1925.

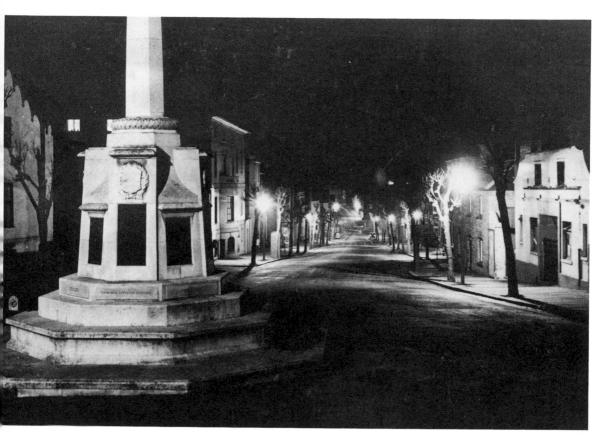

50 This was one of several pictures taken, if I remember correctly, to show the effect of street lighting by new gas lanterns and columns.

Bridge Street

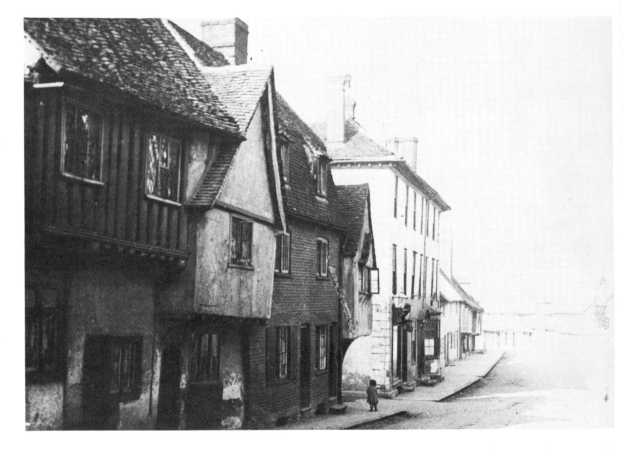

51   *Circa* 1920. Nos 5, 7, 9, 11. Henry Hart, in his *Biographical Notes*, written in 1883 when he was aged 82, recorded in his list of 'Residents whom I have known since 1814' the name 'Nockall. Manager of Silk or Crape Works (Grout & Co) Bridge Street. (About 900 Looms in Walden and surrounding Villages. This brought a considerable amount of Business to the Town.)'

There were so few places in Bridge Street where such a business could have been carried on, that it is conceivable he could have lived at Bridge House (No 15).

Freshwell Street

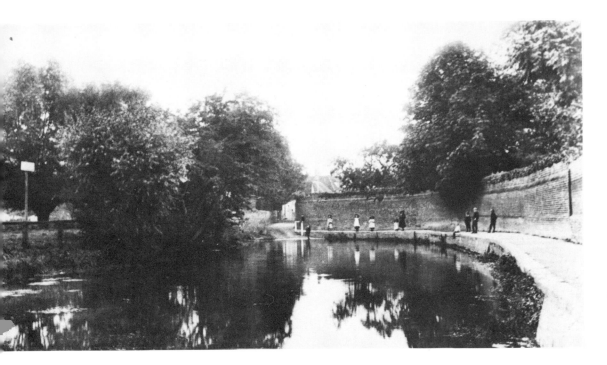

52 New Pond before it was ruined soon after the 1914–18 War. A road had to be made round the outer side of the pond so that motor vehicles could drive through when it was necessary to connect with Freshwell Street or Park Lane.

We boys spent many happy hours sitting on the side like the little boy is doing in the picture, fishing for tiddlers, finding our worms along by the far left-hand wall. We called it 'Titchies' Wall because the meadow on the other side of it belonged to Arthur Titchmarsh.

Horses and carts passed through the pond – the wheels had a clean and 'Dobbin' had a drink. The pond over by the trees was deep and drivers avoided going too close.

Occasionally a small fair would be held in 'Titchies' Meadow when the Common was not available. If the weather was bad, the ground was soon a quagmire. The water level in the Swan Meadows is very near the surface.

53 The 16th-century cottages in Freshwell Street forming the eastern end of Jones' Yard. By 1950 it had changed its name to *Freshwell Gardens*.

The first house in the picture was occupied in boyhood days by Mr Henry Hockley who worked in the nearby livery stables of Dick Williams.

The two rows of houses faced each other. The Yard was entered through the double gates seen in the picture. The houses on the right-hand side had no gardens in front. Those on the left did. At the open west end were more gardens which probably went with the houses on the right facing south.

The far end house was saved from demolition. It was here that Joe Byatt, who lived at 95 Castle Street, had his cobbler's shop. Joe's door can be seen just to the right of the lamp-post. The rough brick floor where Joe worked was about a foot below ground level. Light came from the window under the overhang. I do not know whether Joe also rented the room over or whether it went with the adjoining house.

Joe had one short leg and walked with a simple broomstick crutch. He always went to and from work via Castle Street with a black leather bag under his arm which he used to deliver work done or pick up new work to be done from customers who would look out for him. Joe was part of the Castle Street life of pre-1914 days.

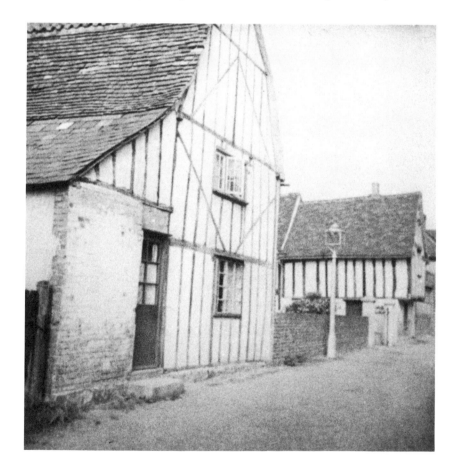

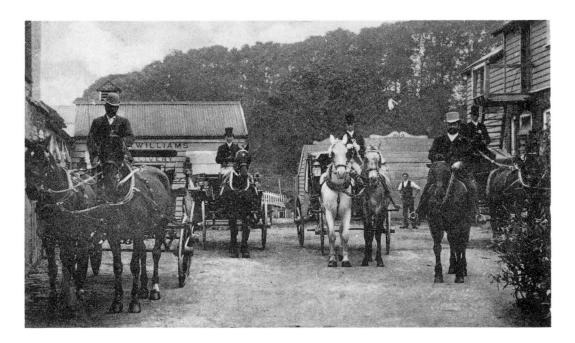

54 Freshwell Street 1905. Richard Atkinson Williams, Jobmaster and Livery Stables, Telephone 011. *Carriages left to right:* 1. Bill Marking, 2. Frank Port, 3. Tom Phillips, 4. H. Hockley. Mr Williams on horseback. R. A. W. was a good cornet player as a young man, and was a member of the Town Band.

Myddylton Place

55   This picture was taken early in the 1914–18 War when Thomas E. Barcham had his grocery and provisions shop at the corner of Myddylton Place. The warehouse was at the rear of the shop with a loading platform opening into Myddylton Place. The horse and cart is probably coming from there after being loaded with orders for delivery to the villages.

Mr Woolnough and Bill Taylor of 17 Debden Road (he later worked at the International Stores) were Barcham's assistants. The shop was No 1 High Street and the Barcham's private house, adjoining, was No 3.

The soldier is posting a letter in the letter-box built into the corner of the wall of the pork butcher's shop, then Tom Wright, later to pass into the hands of Tom Goddard. The Post Office put the box there as a result of pressure from the people living in this part of the town when we had a postal service we could be proud of.

This picture was taken before the east end of what is now the Youth Hostel was stripped of its plaster to expose the timbers.

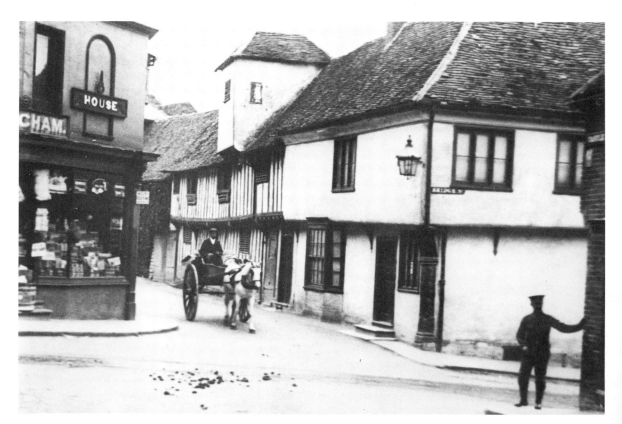

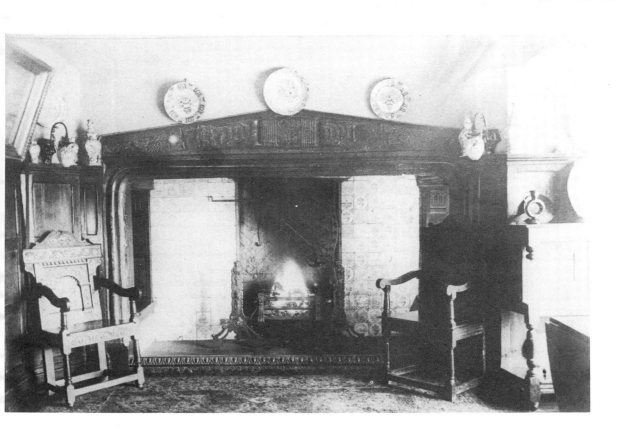

56 The ancient Mantelpiece in Myddylton House. In my History of Hoggs Green (*Antiquarian Society Journal* in the Town Library) I have concluded that this 'Mantle Peice' described by the Society of Antiquaries in 1758, was in the original home of the Myddyltons, called 'Hoggs Green House', a property bequeathed to the almshouses and later sold to George Nicholls, Recorder, who died possessed of it in 1605.

The learned Society's description significantly states that the mantelpiece 'was found in the house of Mrs Elizabeth Fuller and is now placed over her kitchen chimney'. Actually the occupier was *Miss* Elizabeth Fuller, who was left the property by her father, Thomas, who died in 1752. All the evidence suggests that because this ancient mantelpiece is in *Myddylton House*, that property has taken upon itself a history to which it is not entitled but which belonged to the *Hoggs Green House*, demolished *circa* 1758.

A 'John Hogge' witnessed a deed in 1346 relating to a house in 'Hoggsgreene'. 'Hoggs', therefore, did not originate with pigs.

London Road

57 *Circa* 1880. In 1819 a young solicitor's clerk, John Dane Player, son of Joseph Player and a cousin of 'Gentleman' John Player (Mayor 1835), broke away from the Abbey Lane 'Independents' and formed his own 'Particular Baptists' group who met 'in a private house' in High Street.

By 1822, Player and his followers, were able to build their own place of worship in London Road (shown in this picture on the left).

John Dane Player was born in 1800 and died in 1850. Only 19 when he left Abbey Lane, he eventually qualified as a solicitor.

It was John (1839–84), one of his six children, who founded the famous Nottingham Tobacco Co of 'Players' and it was J. D. P.s grandson (also named John Dane Player) who was made an Honorary Freeman of the Borough of Saffron Walden in 1932.

During the Second World War, the chapel was sold and became the headquarters of the Air Training Corps. After the war, the Christian Scientists worshipped there. Some years ago it was converted by Colonel Windle to a private house. The first John Dane Player was buried in the burial ground attached and Freeman J. D. Player restored the memorial stone. Although I appealed to the owner who had the house after Mrs Windle moved, to preserve the memorial stone, it has been moved from its original position, if not destroyed.

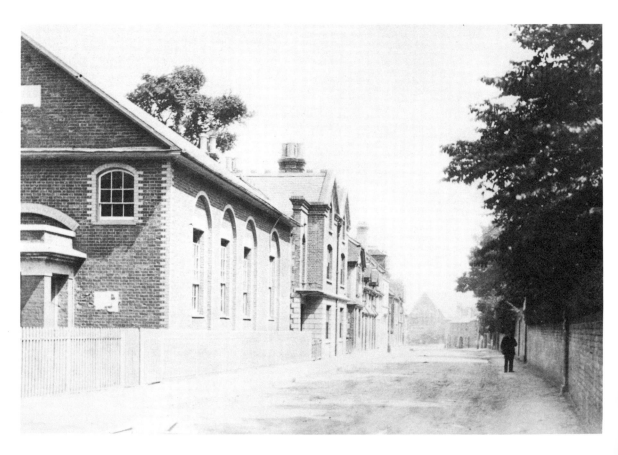

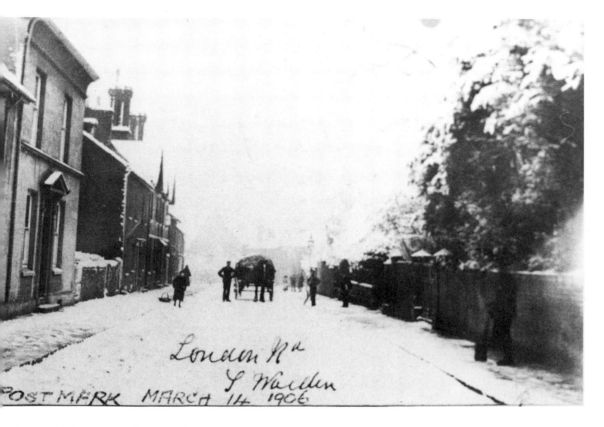

London R^d
Y Warden
POSTMARK MARCH 14 1906

58 1906. There used to be a Good Rule and Government Bye-law which required householders to clear snow from the paths outside their houses by a stated time in the morning. Failure to do so rendered the householder liable to prosecution and a fine.

It was usual at these snowfalls for men, unemployed, to call at houses with offers to clear snow with shovels for a small charge.

The bye-law relating to the clearing of footpaths, fell into disuse because fast-moving motor vehicles splashed back on to the pavements the snow swept into the gutters.

59 *Circa* 1900. Note the sub-post office on the left-hand side. In 1900 the Misses E. and M. Drayton, dressmakers, were there but by 1902 Ellen Cowell, also a dressmaker, was there. William Cowell lived next the post office (where the girl is at the door) and it was behind the glass panel above the door of this house, I believe, that there was always displayed a Bible text.

No 27, *The Orchard*, on the opposite side of the road (behind the brick wall) became the home of Town Clerk William Adams, by 1902. In 1900 he was living in Market Hill.

The Corporation dustcart stands outside *The Lindens*, then occupied by Henry George Brown, a Councillor 1901–13, Alderman 1913–23. By 1904, Mr Brown had moved to 40 South Road, probably when that house was newly built.

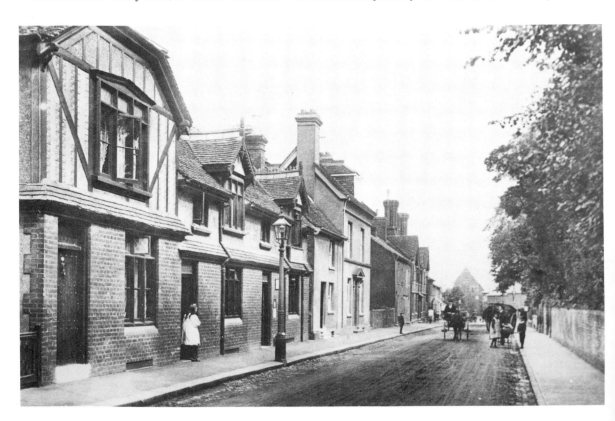

Audley Road

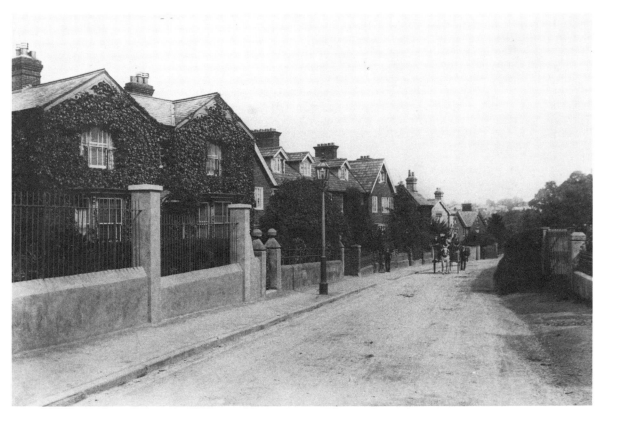

60 Pre-1914. The wall and railings on left continued off the picture with a gate in the centre. It was at the end of the garden made to exhibit plants, etc, behind the nursery of James Vert and Son, which extended from East Street to Audley Road.

Before the houses were built on the right-hand side of Audley Road, Vert also had the large field through the gate shown in the picture, where he grafted fruit trees, budded roses for sale and cultivated it as part of the nursery.

The pair of houses behind the low railing on the right of the picture were built in the late 1890s and were occupied by Charles Tester Parsonage (No 24) and John Reed (No 26). John Reed was the father of Charles Reed with whom I worked at Collin and Adams' office.

James Vert was head gardener at Audley End for Lord Howard de Walden. When Lord Howard left there, Mr Vert went into the nursery business on his own account. When he died, his son, Fred, continued the business but he died a comparatively young man, leaving a widow and three children. Mrs Vert acquired No 62 High Street and ran it as a boarding house, calling it 'Clifton House'.

Debden Road

61   The junction of Debden Road and London Road being widened in 1904. Charles Barker, a jobbing builder of 10 Castle Street, tendered to purchase and remove all buildings for £12 and it was accepted.

Charles Barker stands on the high part of the platform where the wall is being built, George his son, stands next to him and Billy, another son, is fifth in the row. Archie Forbes, the surveyor, stands in the centre with the bowler hat. The Council did the road construction work. Three plane trees were planted here by the Council.

On the left, behind the brick wall, was 'Hockley's Yard', comprising a row of cottages extending behind the first few Debden Road cottages. Hockley's Yard was declared a slum clearance area about 1936, the Yard cleared and the displaced families re-housed.

Daniel Hockley was a builder-architect who was once with William Robinson, the uncle of Henry Hart, and the yard probably took his name because he owned the property.

J. E. Galley, the photographer, and George Golding next door to him are the two shops in London Road looking up Debden Road.

Jim Pateman, butcher, and Owen Baker, grocer, had the two shops on the right of Debden Road, where stands the young man in the white apron.

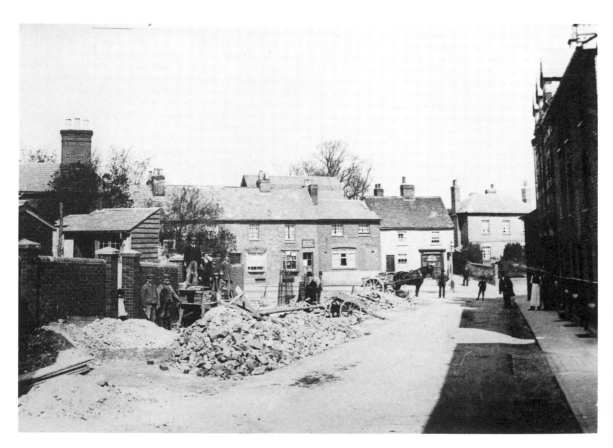

Mount Pleasant Road

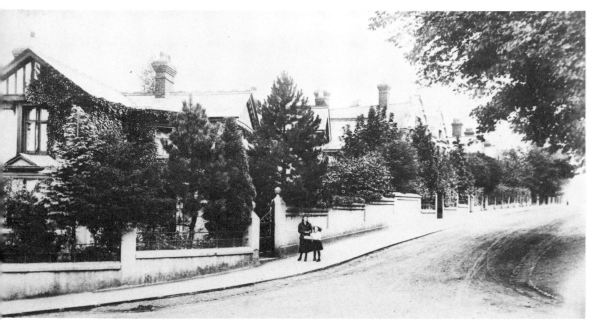

62 *Circa* 1905. When the Friends' School was built in 1879, there were no houses on the north side of Mount Pleasant Road. By 1887 there were about ten residents and the former 'Mill Lane' renamed Mount Pleasant Road. One of the first houses built was 'Saffron Lodge', No 11, the home of Mr W. C. G. Bell, the builder.

   In boyhood days, most people called the road 'Top Road'. The picture shows on the south side, a gutter and an unpaved footpath.

Radwinter Road

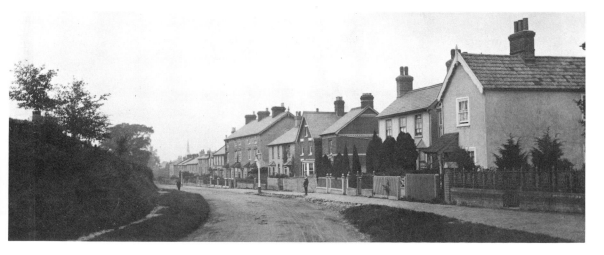

63 *Circa* 1910 before it was paved. The boy in the picture is the photographer's son. Horace Mansell was in business at this time which helps date the picture.

   C. G. Engelmann had not been long at his Horneybrooke Nurseries, entrance to which was between the lamp-post and the boy.

Mandeville Road

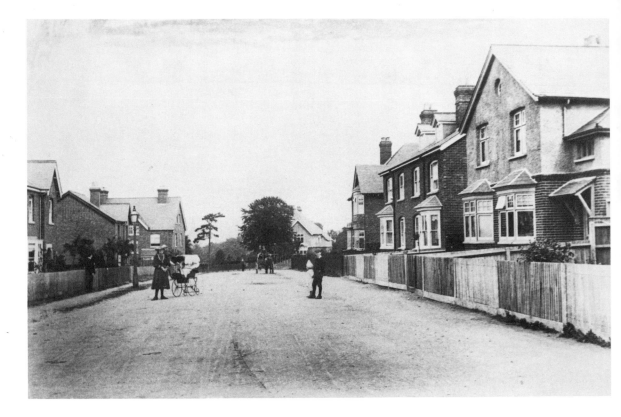

64 The houses in this road were built by Dick Dix commencing about 1906–07. This picture would have been taken about 1912 before it was 'made up' and before *Carclew* was built at far Borough Lane corner.

Civic Amenities

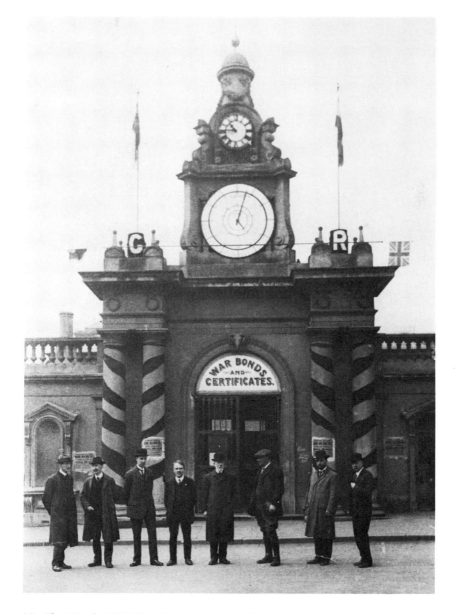

65 The March 1918 War Savings Week at the library. Left to right (War Savings Committee): A. H. Forbes (Borough Surveyor), Guy Maynard (Museum Curator), Samuel Wenman (Hon Treasurer), Hubert Collar (Hon Secretary), Addy Nunn Myhill (Mayor), Peter Giblin Cowell, David Miller, C. H. Youngman (Manager, Barclays Bank). £63,400 raised, 4–9 March inclusive. Arthur Shepherd stands before his office door far right.

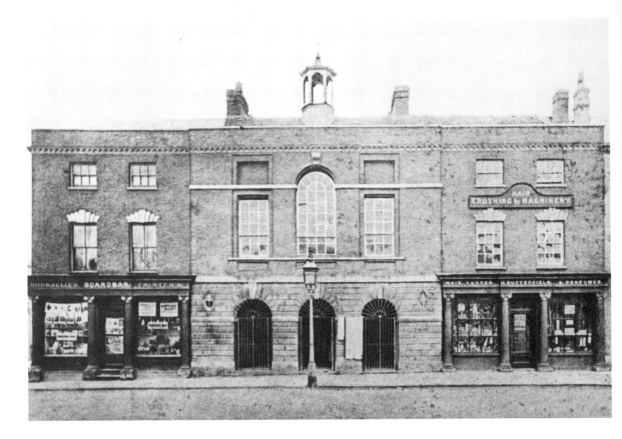

66 Town Hall 1761–1879. Foundation stone laid 15 July 1761.

The shop on the left was originally occupied by George Youngman, Printer, Bookseller, etc. The business passed to his son John Mallows Youngman who sold it to Boardman of Bishop's Stortford.

The barber's shop passed to Burningham after Butterfield; then to W. Windwood, J. T. Pope, H. Startup and then the Westminster bank took a lease of the premises to extend their adjoining premises.

The widow of George Butterfield, hairdresser, died at the New Almshouses on 18 January 1892, aged 80 years. The widow of Henry Butterfield, hairdresser, died aged 86 at her residence in Market Street.

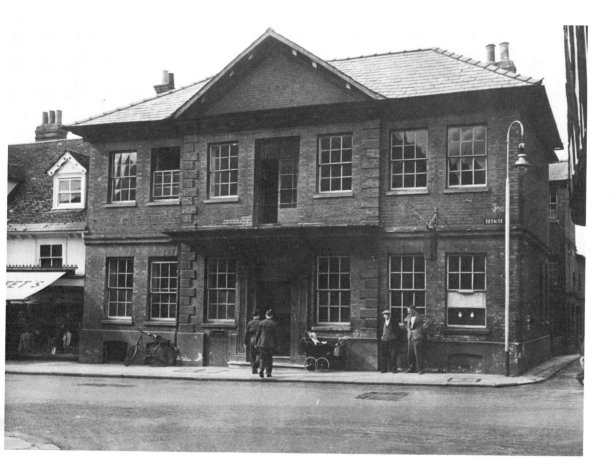

67 High Street – Post Office opened *circa* 1919. The post office as it was *circa* 1940. (Charles Flack and Stanley Mallion by window.) The picture shows Ernest Street's draper's shop on the south side before fire destroyed the property in the 1960s. The shop window, with blind over, used to be the residential end of the property when Mr Street himself had the shop and lived in the house part. A later owner (J. Wandless) extended the shop by taking in the ground floor private house.

The post office was the home of Dr J. P. Atkinson Snr from the time he bought the property in 1881 up to his death in 1917. Dr Atkinson bought the property from William Thurgood who resided in the house. Thurgood was a Solicitor and Clerk to the Justices, 1836 to 1886, and had his office in a cottage behind his house, but in Park Lane.

A Manorial Rental of 1620 shows that *The Swanne Inn* stood on the site and that Park Lane at that time was *Fullers Lane*.

68 Hill Street Swimming Bath and Slipper Baths, opened 29 May 1910. The Slade passes under the enclosed area where the two trees are growing. Miss Gibson presented 2 or 3 cottages for demolition to provide the site of the Baths.

Soon after the Bath was built, the Boys' British School went there in parties on Thursdays when the re-fill water was cold but clean. The water was changed twice a week. We paid a penny, the school a penny and we took our own towel and trunks. Teachers Strong and Hewlett taught us to swim. The Bath was a great improvement on the dirty river at Sir Joshua's Bridge off the Wenden Road!

There was no mixed bathing for some time, but special days and times for ladies. Before the 1914–18 War, two girls thrilled the onlookers at the Water Sports by swimming a length of the baths. They were Maud Baker of Oxborrow's Yard and Hilda Faircloth who eventually married Jack Swan. Both girls during the war, donned PO uniforms to take the places of Percy Pettitt and Gordon Wooldridge the telegraph boys who went to the war.

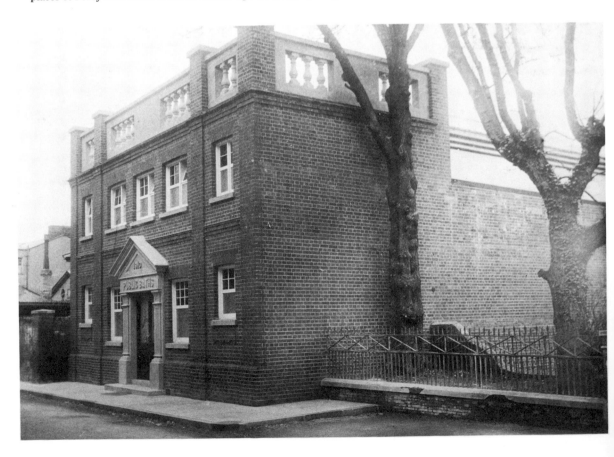

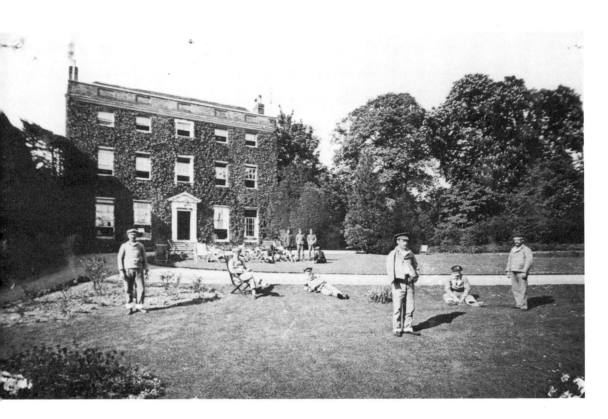

69 Walden Place, Red Cross Hospital 1914–18 War. Occasionally, a local wounded 'Tommy' would be sent from one hospital to his home town and from the many pictures I have of the casualties who were at Walden Place, I have selected this one because there are three wounded Walden men in the group; George Kidman, Harry Perry and Corporal – Downham (Pleasant Valley).

Fred Erswell, Reg Holmes from Alpha Place, 'Mont' Parkin of Wenden, Geoffrey Searle (Wm Adam's Gardener), – Goodwin (Castle Street, Gas Works Stoker) were nursed at Walden Place, some attending after discharge from the army. Many men who were convoyed direct from France had terrible shrapnel wounds.

70 Isolation Hospital *circa* 1902, built in Isolation Lane, later to be called Hill Top Lane. The Scarlet Fever block is on the left. The Matron's house and administration block is on the right. The Diphtheria block was well behind the Scarlet Fever block.

The elderly lady seated is the matron, Mrs Hern and her husband stands behind. (Not to be mistaken for Mr and Mrs Harry Hurn). In the centre of the group is Nell Start, servant and ward maid. The boy in front of her is Ralph Porter who gave me this picture. Also in the group are Winnie Beech, Marjorie and Cynthia Bartlett and Hubert Ridgewell. The pram was presented by Dr H. C. Bartlett. Mrs Sam Cope followed Mrs Hern and she was succeeded by Mrs Henry Poyser.

When I was a scarlet fever patient about 1910, patients received no visitors in the hospital. We had to stand by the iron railing and talk to our parents across the garden through an opening in the corrugated iron fence. The 'Fever Van' (Ambulance) was kept at the hospital and the fumigator was worked by the Matron's husband.

Scarlet fever, common amongst children before World War I and into the 1930s, is scarcely heard of today. Diphtheria, of course, was much much more serious, but medical science has pretty well mastered that disease too. We spent about six weeks in isolation and after about a fortnight in bed feeling ill, the treatment was daily hot baths to assist 'peeling'. We had to lose our old skin and grow new, apparently.

The hospital was administered by the Saffron Walden Joint Hospital Board (Clerk – Wm Adams). I attended meetings, kept the accounts, etc, for some years before I left Mr Adams' service in 1935.

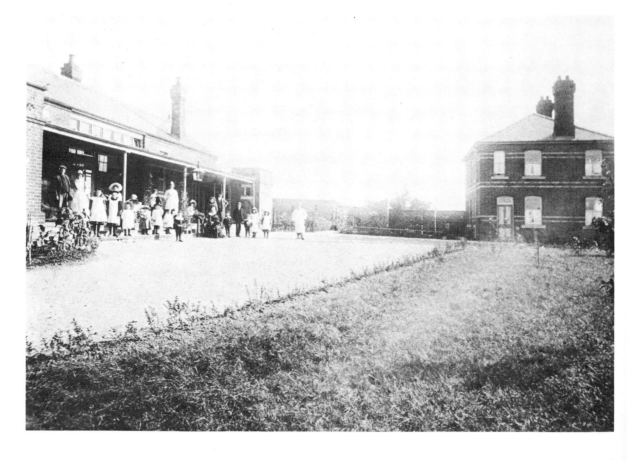

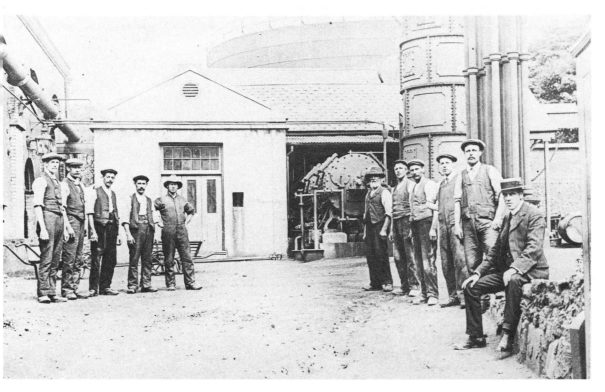

71 Gas Works, Thaxted Road, Staff 1912/13. *Left to right:* John Goodwin, Ted Miller, W. Carter, Jim Reed, Horace Braybrooke, George Westwood, Jim Bacon, Horace Westwood, Frank Day (killed 1914–18 War), Walter Pettitt, George Portass (Manager).

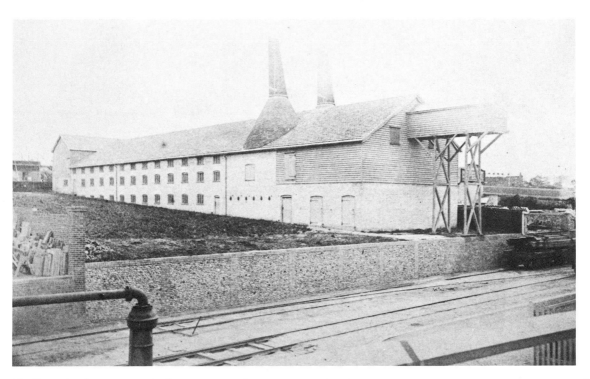

72 West Road – Opposite Railway Station. The Cement Works of Dix, Green & Co. Dick Dix, the grandfather of Arthur, Len and Ralph Dix, also owned the cement works above. Crafton Green, I was told by Len Dix, was a partner with a large financial interest. 'Dix, Green & Co' were included in the Directories for 1887–1907.

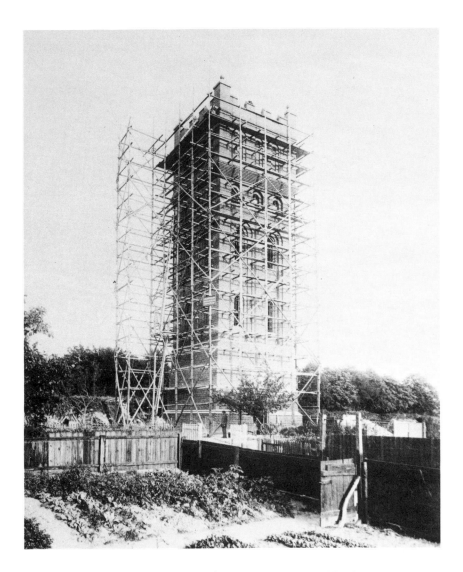

73 The Water Tower in Debden Road. Foundation stone laid by the Mayor, Dr J. P. Atkinson Snr., 9 May 1913. Builder – Jos Custerson, seen in picture at foot of corner scaffolding. Architect and designer – A. H. Forbes, Borough Surveyor.

The tower is 90 feet above ground, 8 feet in the ground. 32,500 bricks were used and 140 tons of concrete. For scaffolding about 500 poles and 1,500 lashes (S. Wenman's note), a scaffolder's work of art before the days of tubular scaffolding.

My father, employed by J. Custerson for many years, worked on the water tower during its construction. He always reckoned that Bob Wilson of Gold Street was the best scaffolder on the staff.

Jack Reed, foreman and principal bricklayer, is standing on the top corner platform. Inside the tower is a winding iron staircase to the reservoir tank and out on to the top of the tower

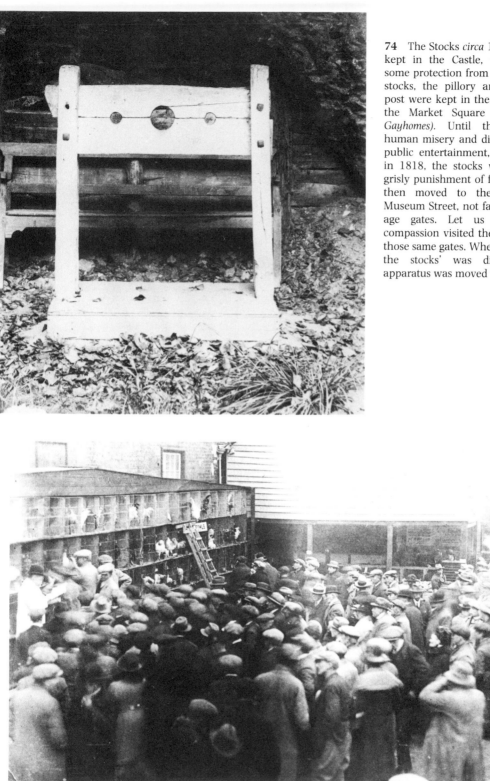

74 The Stocks *circa* 1910. At this time kept in the Castle, where they had some protection from the weather. The stocks, the pillory and the whipping post were kept in the Market Cross on the Market Square (about opposite *Gayhomes)*. Until that platform of human misery and disgrace, venue for public entertainment, was demolished in 1818, the stocks were part of the grisly punishment of felons. They were then moved to the wide area of Museum Street, not far from the Vicarage gates. Let us hope Christian compassion visited the victims through those same gates. When punishment 'in the stocks' was discontinued, the apparatus was moved to the Castle.

75 Borough Market, Hill Street (see also plate 76). Ernest Jennings, Auctioneer, selling poultry at a Tuesday market. (Second left Bob Ridgwell from Bridge Street; extreme right – Mr Bouch and in front of him Harold Westwood.)

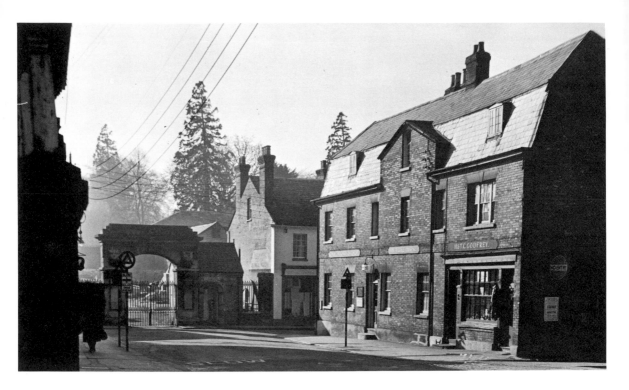

76 Market Street *circa* 1950 showing *White Horse* and Borough Market. The gentlemen's toilet was not there when the Market was constructed originally. I believe it was erected during the time Mr A. H. Forbes was Borough Surveyor (1898–1936).

No 11 Hill Street has been a plumber's, painter's and decorator's shop for many years. Frederick Thorn followed Alfred Rogers there about 1910. I have always understood that this was the 'private house' lent to the Saffron Walden Natural History Society when that body was constituted by Jabez Gibson in 1832, for use as a Museum for the specimens collected by the Society. Jabez Gibson, when he first married, lived in the former Municipal Offices. Then he built *Elm Grove* and lived there. No 11 Hill Street could well have belonged to Jabez Gibson.

The name 'Pig Market' adopted by the District Council is misleading as it gives the impression that the market here is limited to pigs. It never was (see plate 75). The *Borough Market* property, to give it its correct name, was erected in 1831 because the Corporation realised that their 1514 Charter granted them not only market rights and privileges, but imposed, too, responsibilities in the exercise of those rights. The public subscribed £950, negotiated purchase of the land and the *Eight Bells* then standing on it, obtained a tender to build the Market and then handed over the money to the Council, requesting them to complete the job.

The *White Horse*, which has retained its name since 1687 and possibly before that, is built in part over the King's Ditch (later called the Slade) which continued as an open water-course from the Common to the western boundary of the New Almshouses until it was built over in 1832. The name *Market Bridge* by the *White Horse* referred to the bridge over the King's Ditch. The property adjoining the *White Horse* on the west was called *The Bear*.

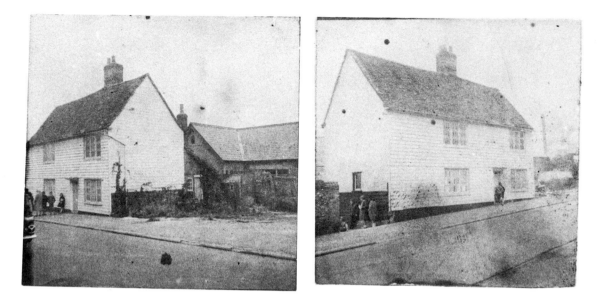

77 This was the School House in Castle Street attached to the National School, demolished in 1966. From 1878 until his death 3 May 1892, Mr Wyndham Butt was the Headmaster. Many Waldenians of my generation will remember Stanley Butt who was born in this schoolhouse (and his twin brother too) on 26 February 1883. Stan wrote to me in 1957: 'The room on the left of the entrance contained oak linenfold panelling. It was afterwards removed and some of it, I believe, went to the Museum in Saffron Walden. I remember there was an exposed beam in the small spare room upstairs. It was used as support for a swing for us boys.' After Headmster Butt died, the schoolhouse was converted into a workshop for boys and a Cookery School for girls. This was done to satisfy the Authorities which, in 1891, were advocating Technical Education in schools.

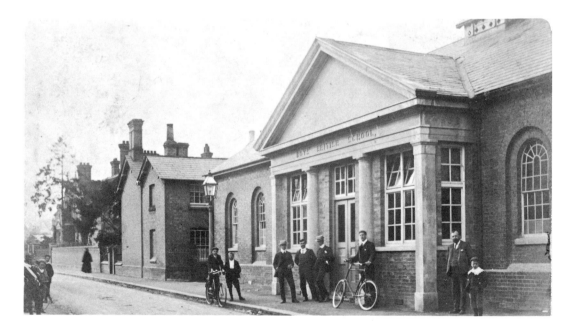

78 East Street – 1906. Boys' British School built 1838. C. Wood, Stanley Hayes, R. A. Strong, E. J. Hewlett (with bicycle), H. Hayes (Headmaster 1891–1924).

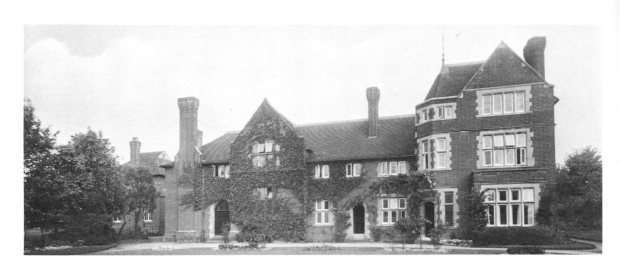

79 Grammar School – Ashdon Road, Built 1881. The School was founded by Charter dated 1525, granted to Dame Jane Bradbury, sister of John Leche, Vicar of the Parish from 1489 to 1521 and whose wish it was to establish the School. The 1525 grant provided that the school curriculum, should be 'after the ordre and use of teching gramer in the Scholes of Wynchester and Eton'. The school was actually started before 1525 under Sir William Dawson, 'a profound Grammarian', in some property he acquired behind what today is 35 Castle Street.

As far as I am aware, a detailed history of the school has not been written. Alderman Rowntree devoted Chapter IX of 'Then and Now' to it, but at the time he wrote, the Grammar School records had not been deposited with the Borough Council. In 1928 a *Short History of the Saffron Walden School 1317–1928* was published, claiming that 'Saffron Walden School is the oldest institution the town possesses', a claim based on a reference in the Walden Abbey Cartulary in 1317 to 'one Reginald, "Scholemaster of Walden" '.

It is my opinion, based on the records which have come down to us, that this claim to foundation earlier than 1525 cannot be sustained. In 1928 the School was, not for the first time, in financial difficulties, increased by the discontinuance about this time of the special rate contribution made to the School by the Borough Education Committee.

In 1846 the Rev Alfred Enoch Fowler, BA of Queens' College, Cambridge, was appointed Master and he remained in office until 1879. He lived at 67 High Street and it would appear that the School during his time was held in the building next to the Friends' Meeting House at the top of the side entrance of Dr Chalmers' Surgery.

The new School in Ashdon Road was made possible largely because of the liberality of Lord Braybrooke who gave the site and George Stacey Gibson who gave £1,000 towards the Building Fund. In his will, G. S. G. also bequeathed £2,000 to the School.

The Rev R. M. Luckock, MA, succeeded Fowler as Headmaster to open the new School. During World War II the school was requisitioned by the RAF, later to become the headquarters of the 65th Fighter Wing of the United States Army Air Force.

After the war, the school was leased to the Training College and used as a Hostel. Other buildings (Nissen huts) erected in the grounds during the war, were used as a Junior School to become known as Dame Bradbury's School which now has the benefit of the charitable funds of the old Free Grammar School

The Dame Bradbury School was brought into existence largely through the efforts of Mr Frederic B. Malim, Miss M. Gale and Alderman C. B. Rowntree – all educationalists

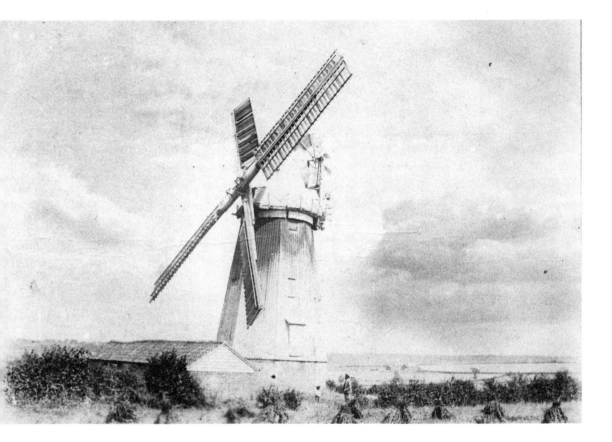

80 This is the Windmill, demolished about 1900 which, according to the 1877 Ordnance Map, stood at the southern end of field No 728 some 200 yards away from Mill House, which still exists on Peaslands Road.

Jim Wright, the last miller, lived in the Mill House, which is now No 18. Brian and Horace, his sons, were school fellows. Jim Wright stood as umpire at cricket matches on the Common. He had been Captain of the Town Club in the 1890s and was recalled about 1902.

In some notes I have of Samuel Wenman's, he records that the windmill 'ceased work 1897 or 1898 and then was pulled down'.

The picture was given to me by Arthur W. Parker, the small boy in the picture, near his father, Arthur Parker, who lived in South Road and was foreman carpenter at the Gibson estate yard in Debden Road. It was Parker himself who told me he judged the date to be about 1900.

The road *Old Mill Road* was named to perpetuate the location of this mill.

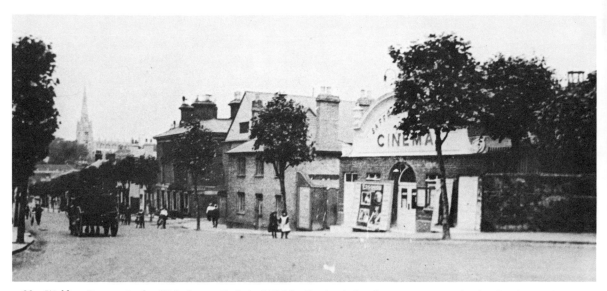

81 Walden Cinema in the High Street. Built in 1912 by Rooke & Son for Ernest E. Smith of Bishop's Stortford. The original cinema was planned so that from the box office in the front, the floor rose rather steeply to a flat gangway separating the higher priced seats at the High Street end from the cheaper seats on the other side of the gangway, the floor of which sloped downwards.

The projector room was at the far end behind the screen. Some time later (after the 1914–18 War) the entire floor was taken out and a new one laid providing an auditorium of 420 seats. The screen was at the High Street end and the floor made to rise from front to back with a gangway across the centre to separate the sheep from the goats! The film was projected over the heads of the audience.

Sergeant Jarman was the attendant when the cinema first opened and in the days of the silent films Miss Freestone was the pianist at one stage. She was the daughter of George Freestone the Engineer of South Road and later married Herbert Taylor of 19 London Road, who was a printer for Blooms.

This was not the first cinema, for Andrew R. Dix opened one in the Central Hall before 1912. On Saturdays there were two evening performances. After the first, starting about 6 pm, the room was cleared and the second show commenced with an entirely new audience. I can remember the matinees starting on Saturday afternoons.

Fire completely destroyed 'The Walden' in 1950. Manager H. J. Langford was away on holiday at the time and chief operator Percy Sutton, after cleaning up about mid-day with everything ready for the evening show at 5 pm went to his adjoining house when he noticed smoke coming from the cinema. The building was largely of timber construction so the fire got rapid hold and was a total loss.

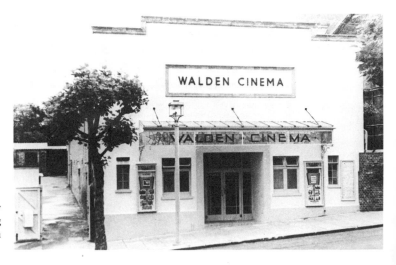

82 This is the frontage of the new cinema built after the above building was destroyed by fire. This new cinema was opened early in 1954.

Railway

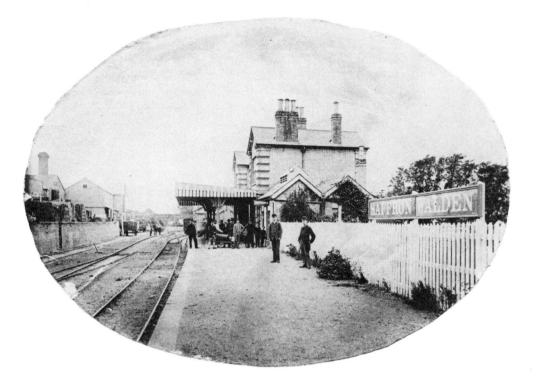

83 The Great Eastern Railway branch line from Audley End to Bartlow, to connect with the Shelford–Marks Tey line, was constructed in the early 1860s

The Audley End–Saffron Walden part of the line was opened on 21 November 1865. That part from Walden to Bartlow was opened on 26 October 1866.

The first train to run on the branch line from Walden to Audley End was the 8.45 on the morning of Thursday, 23 November 1865. Upon that occasion it rained hard. The Town Band, however, played at the station entrance gates in the presence of a considerable number of people. The engine used was No 60, driven by engine driver John Duce who, by 1891, had died. The guard was Charles Newson who in 1891 'still journeys upon the trains as of old'. The original engine had, by the same year, 'gone the way of all things'.

Walden's station was closed to passengers on 7 September 1964 and for all goods traffic on 28 December following.

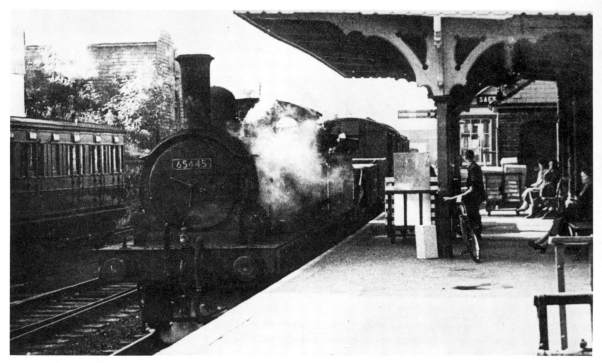

84 Saffron Walden Railway Station.

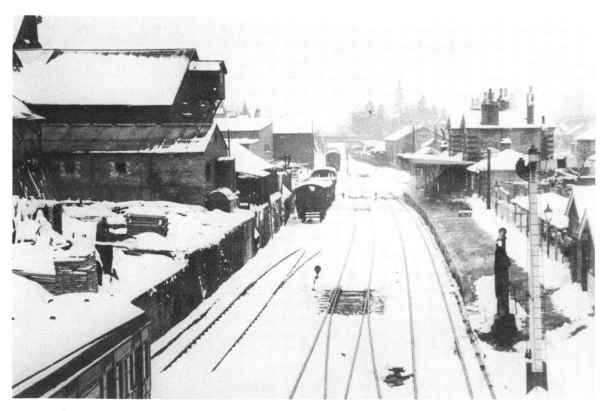

85 Looking out to Debden Road Bridge from the South Road Bridge after a fall of snow. I wonder how many times guard Alfred Sutton stood, watch in hand, at this near end of the platform, looking over to the raised Station Road, to ginger up his season ticket regulars, saving them from getting to work late by missing the mainline train. I would think Mr Sutton knew to a second just how long he could wait before blowing his 'all aboard' whistle. He did many a good turn to the few commuters of his time.

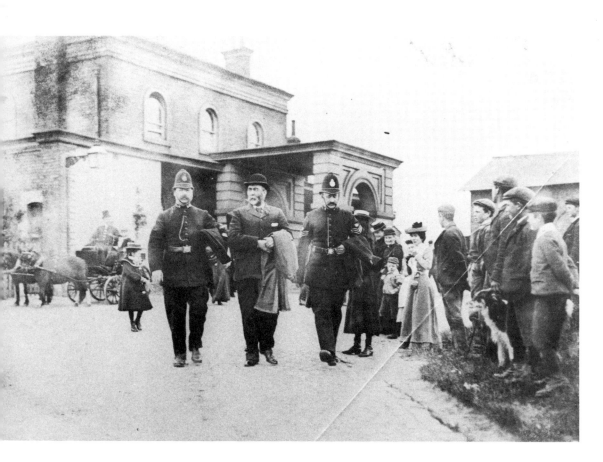

86   Samuel Dougal of the Moat Farm, Clavering and murderer of Miss Camille Holland in 1899.

The murder did not come to light until four years later. He is handcuffed and being escorted from the main line at Audley End to the branch line to appear before the local Petty Sessions. He stood trial at the Chelmsford Summer Assize of 1903 and was found guilty. He confessed to his ugly crime and was hanged in Chelmsford prison on 14 July 1903.

On one occasion when he was kept in a cell at the Walden police station, he took off his diamond ring and scratched his initials on a large panel of glass, part of a glazed screen in the station.

87 Great Eastern Railway Goods Depot Staff about 1912. *Back row:* Wm Munden (horse shunter); Wm Chipperfield (carman) and E. D. Swan (carman). *Second row:* Wm ('Weeley') Housden (carman); H. S. Smith (clerk); Robt Shaw (goods porter); W. Regelous (goods porter). *Seated:* R. Hardy (clerk); S. Brown (goods foreman); E. Blanchfield (station master); H. Gapes (chief clerk); Bert L. Harris (clerk); Fred W. Goddard (junior clerk). *Front:* P. D. Mansfield (shunt horse chain lad); Sidney Newman (junior clerk).

Carman Swan's son, Charlie, also gave many years' railway service as a station clerk. He was Borough Councillor 1958–61 and 1963–68, and a JP. Bill Housden stood as a Labour candidate on 2 or 3 occasions, but was not elected. Fred Goddard became a Councillor, Alderman and Mayor. Percy Mansfield lost a leg in the 1914–18 War, I think, and for several years was a ticket collector on Cambridge station.

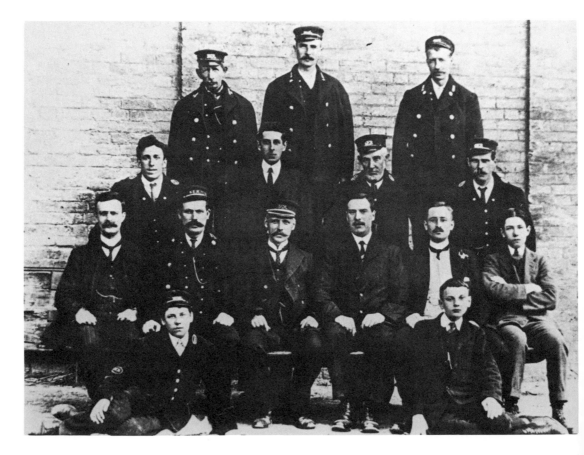

Local Traders

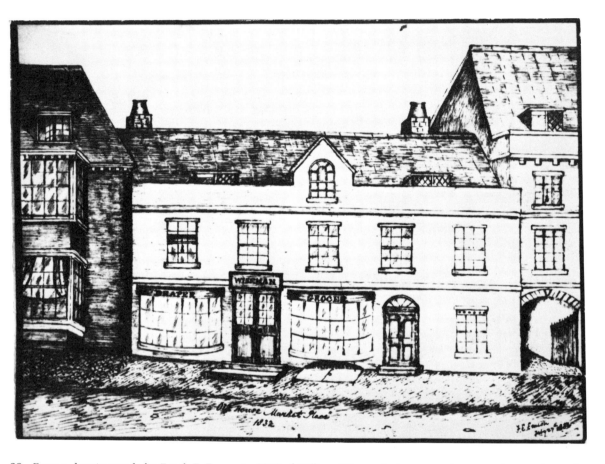

88 From a drawing made by Frank E. Emson in 1882 of William Wiseman's drapery and grocery shop, as it was in 1832 in Market Place. The shop stood on the site of *The Angel Inn* (previously *The Horn*). It might even have been *The Angel*. It was acquired by the Gibsons along with the *Rose and Crown* adjoining, and it was on this site they built their new bank in 1874 after 50 years' business in Market Hill.

The house on the left was built by William Robinson for and occupied by Mr *Gentleman* John Player, Walden's first Mayor under the Municipal Corporations Act, 1835. The garden at the rear extended to the Common.

The building on the right was the ancient *Rose and Crown*. The side passage leading to the yard and stables at the back and on to Common Hill, was retained by Boots when they re-developed the site after the *Rose and Crown* was destroyed by fire at Christmas, 1969.

The first Gibson bank in Market Hill was called *Saffron Walden and North Essex Bank* – now No 13, an antique shop.

89 Henry Hart, born at Linton in 1801, was apprenticed to George Youngman, a printer who had succeeded J. Wallis an artist and bookseller, who occupied what is now 'Winstanley House' in Market Hill opposite the old *Green Dragon* (now Trustee Savings Bank). Hart stayed with Youngman until 1836 when he opened his own business as a Printer, Bookseller, etc, 'in the house opposite' No 18 King Street which would appear to be No 21 King street (late A. H. Gatward, optician).

Henry Hart is shown outside No 18 King Street, which property he took over at some time after 1876 and before he died in 1883. Henry was the grandfather of the W. Ernest Hart old Waldenians will remember as a great pal of Charles Hagger, the antiques dealer. The property adjoining No 18 on the right was a private house of which there is a photograph in the Town Library.

I wonder how long it took to water all those flower pots above the shop windows! They were a feature of the shop front for many years.

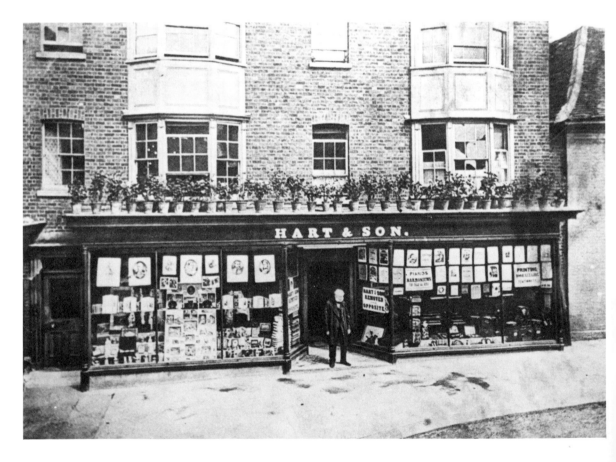

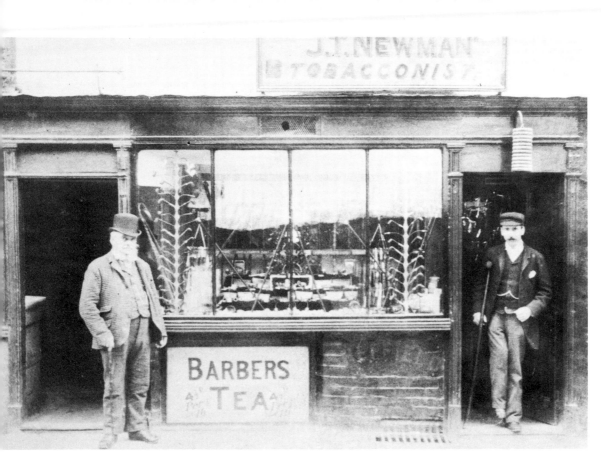

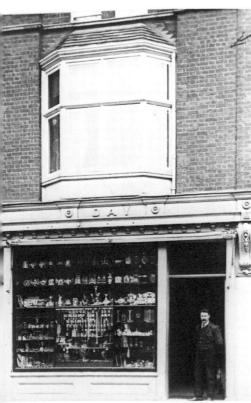

90 No 11 King Street, *circa* 1896. James T. Newman (with crutch) and his father, outside his tobacconist's shop next to Hardwicks. The door on the left is Hardwicks. *Note:* sign over door – a gold painted roll of 'twist' tobaccco, bound and stringed – the Tobacconist's Sign. Price of tea 4½d a ¼lb.

According to an old Directory, Newman's business was established in 1868. The 1887 Directory does not include a Newman under King Street, but it does record 'Rippon, Alfred A., tobacconist', so it would be fair to assume that Newman's shop was previously Rippon's

91 This picture shows Arthur F. James outside the shop, 8 King Street, then occupied by H. W. Day watchmaker and jeweller, his employer. Arthur was the son of John James, a jeweller who had his shop in Cross Street, now Millers. Lime Tree Passage is on the right of picture.

Day found he could not afford the much-increased rent demanded of him and he offered the business and stock to Arthur, his assistant, if he could find other and cheaper premises. With the help of Fred Pitstow Jnr, his wife's nephew, he came to terms with Arthur Titchmarsh for the hire of a front room of the house next to his shop, No 35 King Street. Behind this front room was a smaller one with a skylight, used by a dentist. Arthur James eventually took over this second room for his workshop. It was here that Arthur James taught Len Pitstow, another nephew, the arts and crafts of a watchmaker and jeweller. After his uncle's death Len took over the business.

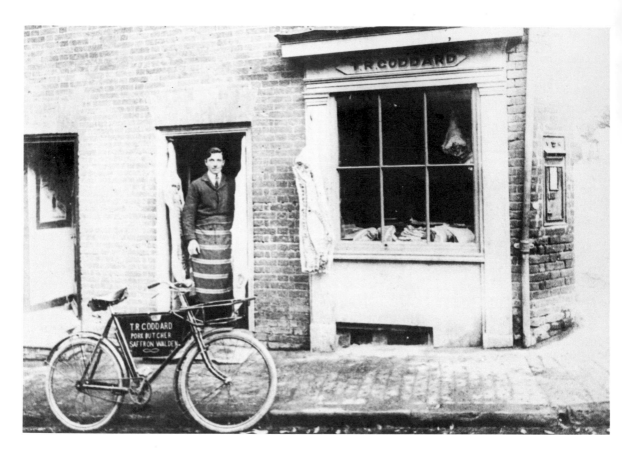

92 In 1904 Ellen Shepherd, Pork Butcher, occupied this property at No 2 Bridge Street. She appears also in the 1892 Directory. She was probably the widow or daughter of William Shepherd who was on the 1881 Burgess Roll for Bridge Street. Tom Wright succeeded her. Shortly after the 1914–18 War, Tom Goddard, who lived with his parents at *The Five Bells*, Castle Street, bought the business when he was in his early 20s. He stands at the entrance to his shop. He built up a good trade and made the best pork sausages in Walden!

By 1933 he had done well enough to buy Hubert A. Britton's butchery business in Church Street with its own slaughterhouse. Tom employed his brothers George, Stan and Reg and in later years, his sons Norman and Richard who now run the business. Tom married Edith Lacey, daughter of Tom, a well-known Waldenian.

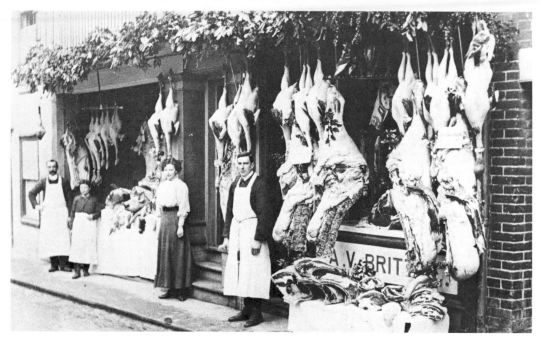

93 Augustus Victor Britton's butcher's shop between the Liberal Club on the left and the *Old English Gentleman* on the right in Gold Street *circa* 1912. *Left to right:* 'Shine' Rushforth, 'Polly' Perkins, Miss Day, A. V. Britton.

A. V. and Hubert A. Britton were sons of D. G. Britton, all butchers. H. A. B. had his business in Church Street (now Goddards).

This picture would have been taken just before Christmas because of the turkeys and greenery displayed. The great carcasses of beef have tickets indicating that the beast won a prize in the Fatstock Market. Mr Britton later moved to the shop at the corner of High Street and George Street, opposite the *Abbey Hotel*, in the occupation of Mr Willett.

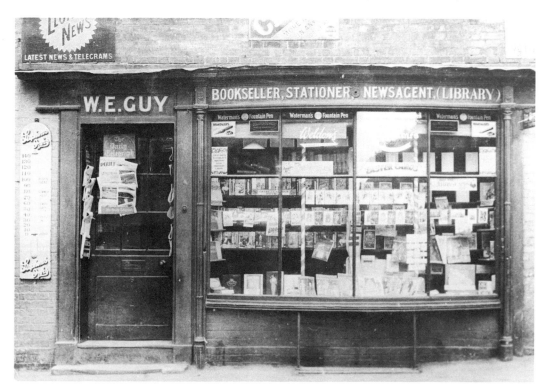

94 The front of W. E. Guy's shop taken about 1920; this is now the Victoria Wine Stores.

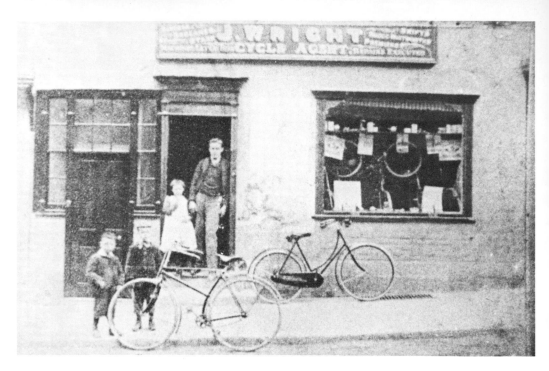

95 This picture was taken about 1899 and shows Mr Joseph Wright, as a young man, standing in the doorway of his cycle shop at 25 High Street with one of his two daughters. No 25 is today the Radio Supply Stores. The door next to Mr Wright's was the private entrance to the living quarters over Cro's Stores (later Housden's)

    In the Directory for 1900, Joe Wright had moved across the street to No 26 where he built a large motor showroom and cycle shop, with a garage and repair shop at the back (site of Woolworths).

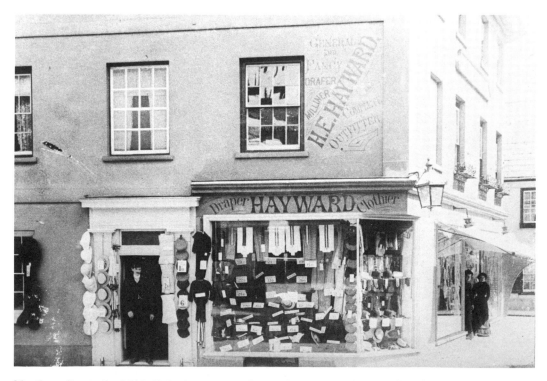

96 Cross Street *circa* 1902. H. E. Hayward standing at the Market Row door of his shop. The two lady assistants stand at the main Cross Street entrance to the drapery department. Round the corner, in Hill Street, was another department and the entrance to his private quarters above the shop.

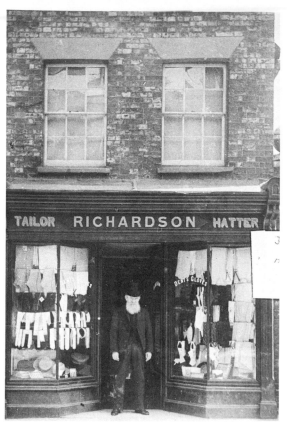

97 W. Richardson, who stands in his shop doorway at 38 High Street, moved here in November 1877, where he had been in business for 15 years (ie from 1862). His advertisement in Hart's 1866 Companion describes him as a 'Tailor, etc, Established 1828 (late Housden)' in Bridge Street. His son, William Rowley Richardson, continued the business. The family lived in Mandeville Road. Mr Richardson Snr made the livery for Lord Braybrooke.

The shop was next to the yard which in later years was developed as the Central Arcade. The shop then was occupied by William E. Armstrong, the watchmaker, before he moved to 31 High Street.

98 Stebbing Leverett's window display in Market Hill, probably during the time Arthur Newman was manager, between the two wars. I remember the Jaeger agency Leverett had and the high quality of the goods of that name.

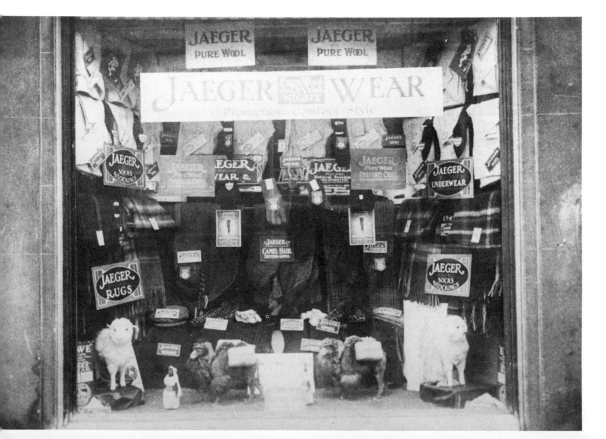

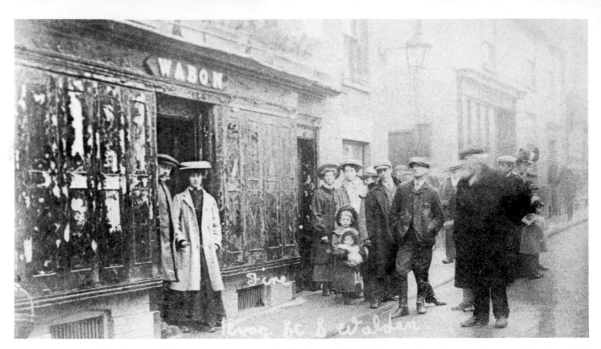

99   Mr R. W. Wabon's sweet-shop at 28 King Street badly damaged by the intense heat from a fire opposite. I was told that the premises destroyed by the fire were at the time in the occupation of Harold Woodward, Auctioneer, who, by 1912 was at 13 Hill Street in business as Woodward and Priday.

It is as a sweet-shop that I remember it, but Wabon advertised himself as in business there as a paperhanger, painter, etc.

Sweets and chocolates were displayed opposite the entrance door on a counter with some kind of framework built on the slope on which the boxes of sweets, without tops, could tickle your fancy. Over the top of the whole display of sweeties, Wabon fixed a frame of ¼ inch mesh wire to stop customers helping themselves! It is that wire which sticks in my memory. Old Reuben Nash who had the sweet-shop opposite the Boys' British School also put wire between customer and goods. It took a long time in those days to spend the rare halfpenny pocket-money and there were 480 of them in the £ of 100 pence today.

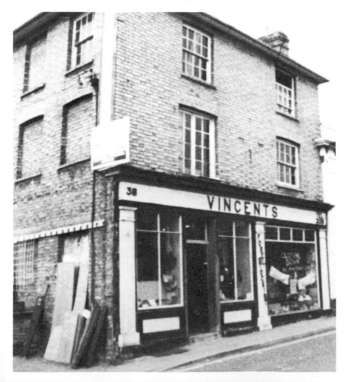

100   Nos 38 and 40 Church Street. Hart's 1893 Directory records that 'Frederic Henry Johnson of Saffron Walden begs to announce that he has purchased all the Ironmongery, Ironfoundry, Engineering and Agricultural Implement business, situate in Church Street, Saffron Walden, hitherto carried on by his brother Thomas Rider Johnson, under the firm or style of "Thomas Johnson & Son" – which business was established by a member of the family, about the year 1810. And that he intends continuing the above business under the same name and in all its departments, as hitherto; he sincerely trusts that, by prompt and careful attention to all orders entrusted to him and by dealing only in goods of the best description at reasonable prices, he may merit and secure the confidence and support of all former customers and the general public.

Church Street, Saffron Walden, March 1892.'

After Johnsons came C. Medcalf & Son, then L. R. Scrimshaw, then Vincents, sadly closed in 1980.

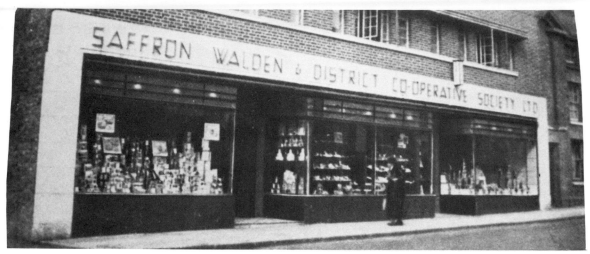

101 Nos 33–35 High Street, present central Co-op, opened 1935.

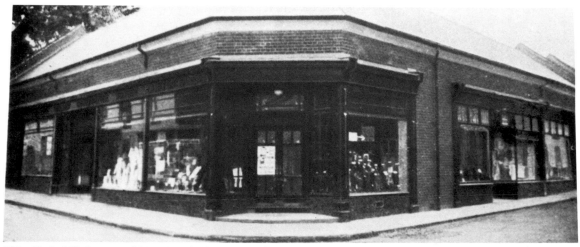

102 No 1 Hill Street and Nos 7–9 Gold Street. Built on the site of the old Liberal Club which the Co-op Society acquired probably just after the 1914–18 War.

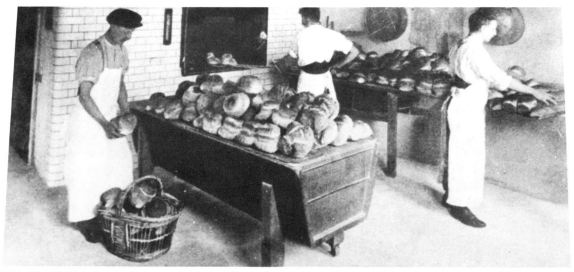

103 No 48 High Street. The new Co-op bakehouse built at the rear of the central premises, opened 1912. Charlie Start; Ted Stock; W. J. (*Scotchy*) Clark.

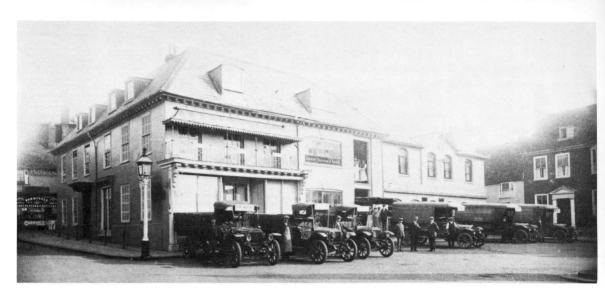

104 Emson Tanner & Sons, Wholesale Grocers, Market Square, where *Gayhomes* now stands. Taken in the early 1920s with the Emson Tanner fleet of lorries outside. 1st lorry – Chas Coe. Centre – E. G. Cornell, E. W. Tanner, John Green.

I think Jack Mumford is the driver standing by his vehicle (last but one). Cecil Sillett is the office boy with the cap, on the warehouse loading platform.

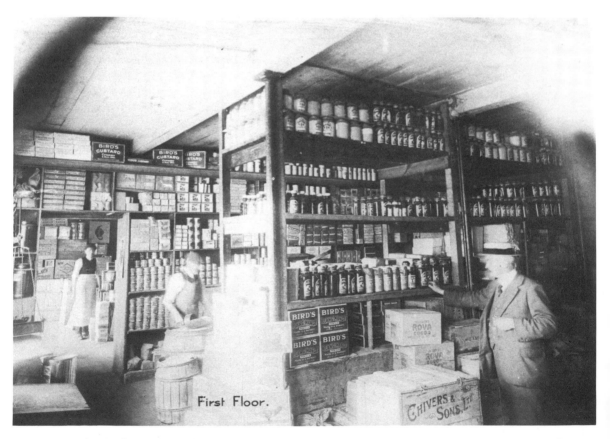

105 Tanner's Warehouse, first floor. Sid Golding; 'Dandy' Richardson; John Green, Manager, who lived in flat over office.

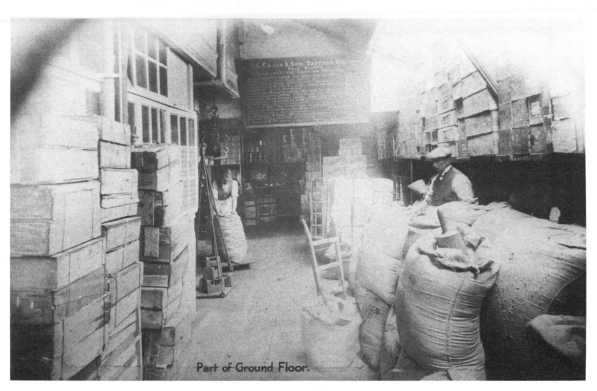

106 Part of Tanner's ground floor warehouse. John Cowell weighing a loaded sack on scales, and Arthur Livett.

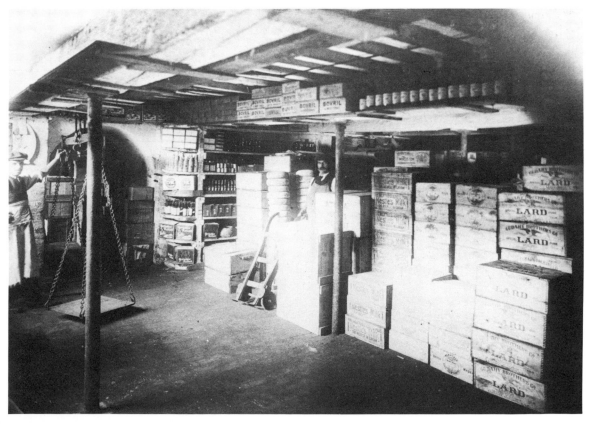

107 In the cellar warehouse of Tanner's. Frank (*Choke*) Bacon by scales. Other employee not known.

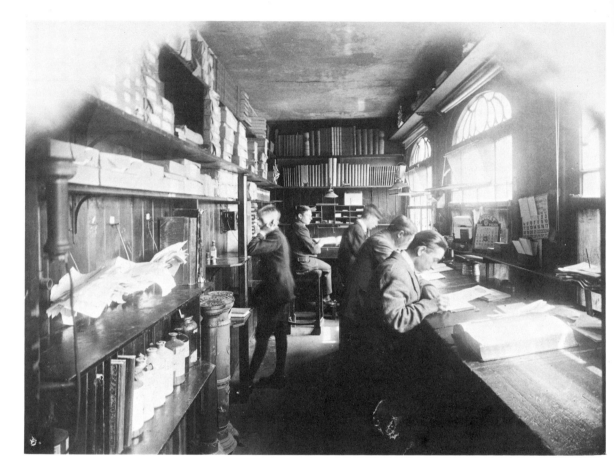

108 Emson Tanner & Sons' office, in the 1920s. Cecil Sillett is on the direct telephone line to Robsons, Station Street. Bert Evenett, back from the War, sits on his stool at the far end. On the right is George Baker, E. G. Cornell and Vic Smith (a cripple from Middle Square).

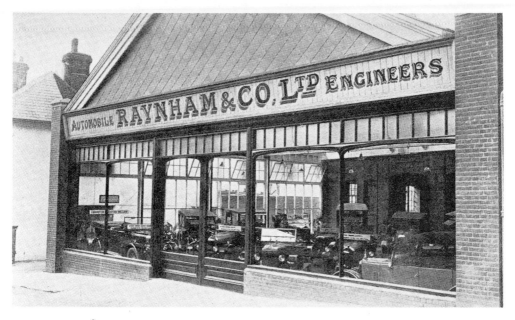

109 This picture shows the finished showroom and through the window can be seen the old brewery loading bays.

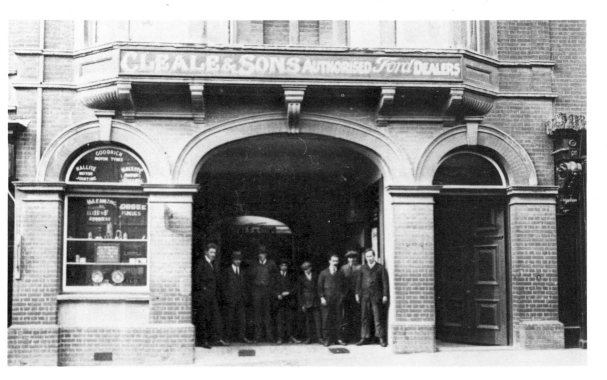

110 The post office moved from King Street to its present situation in High Street about 1919.

The property was taken over by J. W. Whalley of Bishop's Stortford, who set up the business of Cleale & Sons, authorised Ford dealers, about 1920. *Left to right:* Wallis (Manager), John Whalley, – Hadler of Cleale & Hadler, Customer, Boy, Arthur Aves, John Mellor, Harry (*Jot*) Taylor.

Whalley sold the business to Albert Hatch and A. F. Jossaume who, as partners traded as 'Cleales'. The sign 'Cleale & Son' covers 'Saffron Walden Post Office' cut into the stonework. Above the two bay windows is the Royal Arms. Cleales moved to Station Road.

Frank Wright, High Street, was, I believe, the first local Ford agent and A. N. Raynham followed.

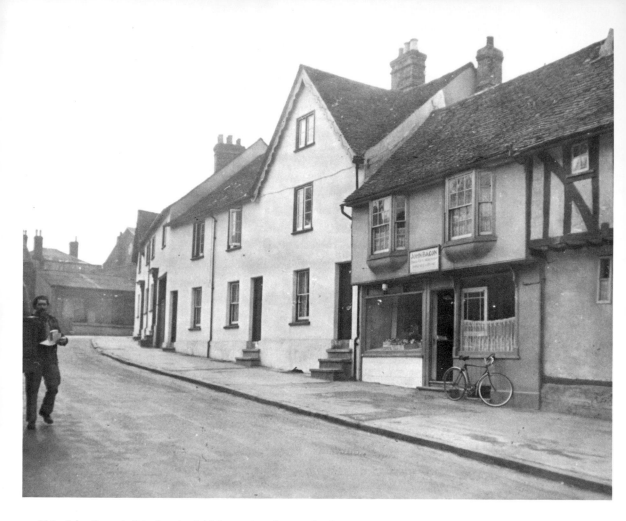

111 John Bacon's fish shop in Gold Street. See plate 24 for the same view in 1843.

The gateway leads to a yard shared by all the tenants. Alf Walls, who lived at No 48, had his cobbler's shop across the yard. The outside WCs were also there.

Churches

112 Parish Church – from Battle Ditches. Engraving between 1811 and 1831. Engraved by T. Higham from a drawing by J. Greig for the *Excursions through Essex*. The drawing must have been made before the church lanthorn was replaced in 1831/32 by the spire and after the Congregational Church was built 1811. The tall building by the church would be Dorset House, the buildings left (west) of the Congregational Chapel would be the 1782 Almshouses demolished in 1950 to make room for the Joseph Prime two-bedroomed bungalows. The meadow in the foreground which contained the Saxon burial ground, later formed part of the Hill House garden and grounds. *Note* the water-bearing ditch on the north and east sides of the raised footpath in Battle Ditches from where the artist made his drawing. The water probably discharged in the pond which was in front of the 1881 West Wing almshouse block, filled in probably when the Slade was arched in 1832 to make room for the New Almshouses built 1834.

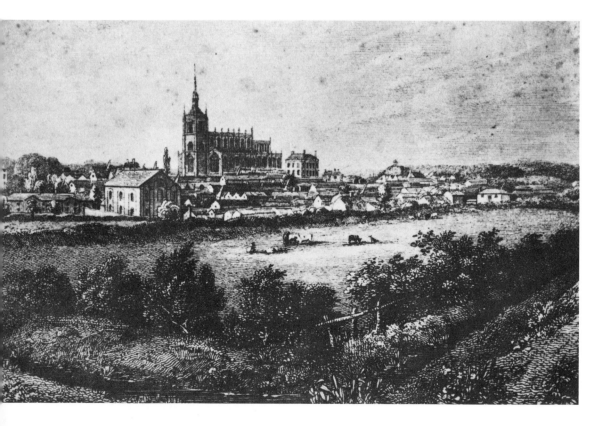

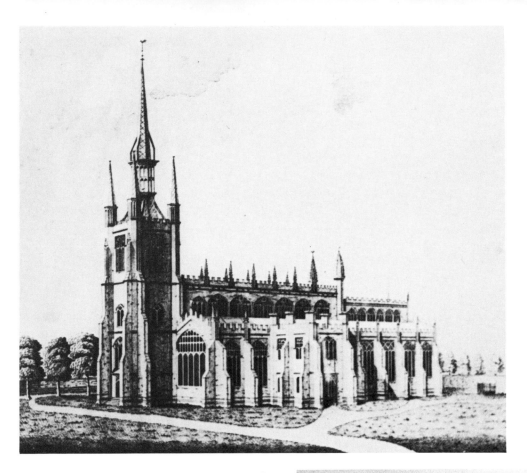

113 An engraving by I. Roberts from a drawing by William Robinson Jnr, made in 1784 of the south-west view of the church. The plate is 'with all due submission dedicated to the Worshipful Mayor, Aldermen and Corporation by their Townsman and Obedient Servant Wm Robinson.'

Robinson was the uncle of Henry Hart, the founder of Harts the Printers. He built the Grove on Chater's Hill in 1804.

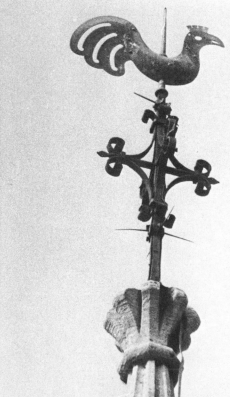

114 The Weathercock on top of the church spire, taken by David Campbell with a long-distance lens.

I heard it said many years ago that during a severe thunderstorm, Wycliffe Leverett, a churchwarden I believe, saw from his house in the Market Place, a streak of lightning strike the steeple and run down to earth by the lightning conductor. One can be seen in this picture.

Steeplejacks went up to the weather cock to inspect the conductor and the state of the spire. I have always understood that it was at this time that the topmost stone and the iron bracket for the weather cock had to be replaced and that it is the old one which is at the foot of the tower, south side, near the west door. I believe the lightning conductor had to be renewed too.

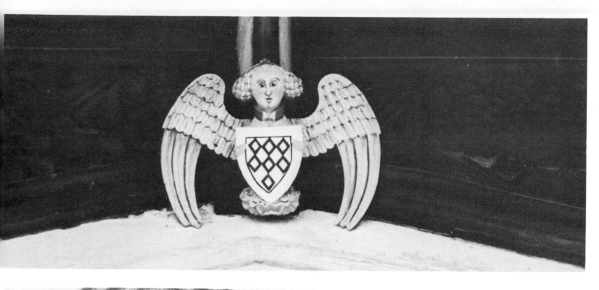

115 One of the bosses in the roof of the nave of the Parish Church. Another picture by David Campbell.

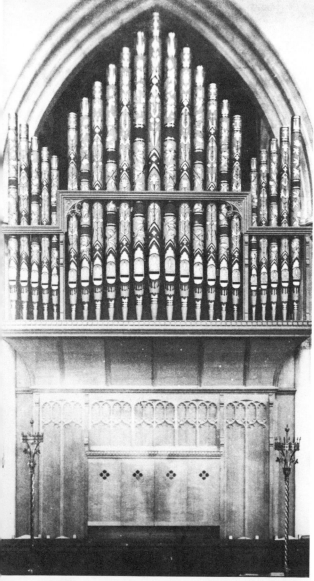

116 Churchwarden, Thomas Frye, launched a scheme in 1822 for the building of an organ which, previously, the church did not possess. John Vincent was the successful tenderer at £497. The money was raised by public subscriptions. Vincent did such a first-rate job, using only the best materials, that he spent £800 on the contract. A further £70 was raised by subscriptions which left Vincent short by £233. It is not clear whether Vincent received any further payment for building the organ, but he tuned it and made minor alterations to it for some years after, so perhaps we may assume he was saved from the ruin with which he said he was faced if the £233 was not paid.

The organ was completed in 1824 and Thomas Frye's son, John Thomas, aged 12, a musical prodigy, was appointed church organist, a position he held until 1884.

The organ was rebuilt in 1885 after J. T. Frye resigned, at a cost of £1,147 and was reconstructed in 1911 at a further cost of £1,127.

Thomas Frye was the Borough Treasurer 1836–50, to be succeeded by his son in 1850 – until he died 23 October 1887.

117 Parish Church. When the rood screen was being made and erected in 1923 (by a Coggeshall firm I believe), I was living in Castle Street, walking every day through the churchyard to work at 14 Church Street. I often looked in at the church in my dinner-hour to see how work was progressing, to admire the craftsmanship of the woodcarvers and to talk with them.

A workman talked to me on one occasion about the memorial stone covering the grave of John Leverett opposite the door of the Parish Room. The name 'Leverett' he had never met before and it so intrigued him that he carved a small leveret on the rood screen. He pointed it out to me at the top left-hand end where the screen joins the stone pillar.

I have told this story myself several times because it was not known officially. Few people notice the baby hare in the position it is and would not be able to account for it if they did. To me, the carver perpetuated a well-known Walden family.

This picture was taken before the rood was added in later years. Lighting was still by gas.

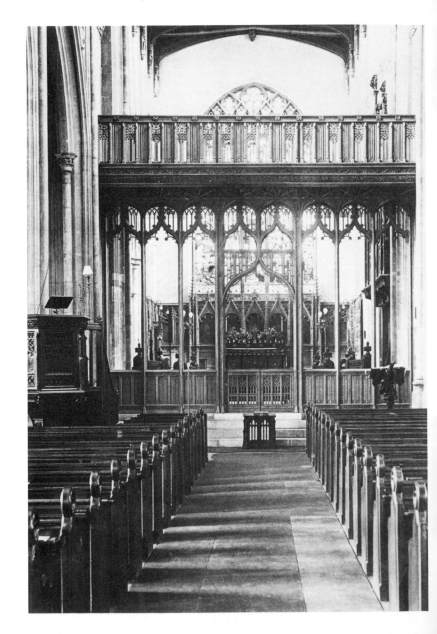

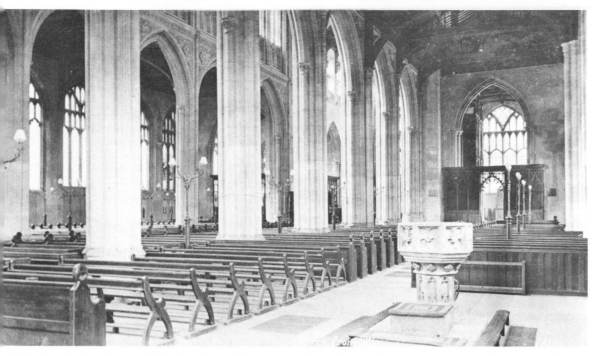

118 Parish Church *circa* 1912. View from SW corner of church by the font looking across to the vestry and north aisle. The font stood, earlier, at the west end of the nave. The church, at this time, is gas lit.

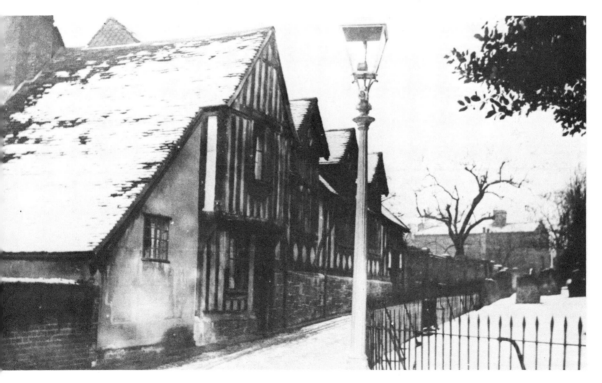

119 Verger's House, Churchyard and Parish Room. Before the Walden Lodge of Freemasons acquired their own premises in Church Street, Lodge meetings were held in the Parish Room. On my way home from school I would occasionally satisfy my curiosity by looking in at the door, George Moss Taylor was the 'Tyler' at the time, Jack Penning his assistant. It is Jack I remember most. The check-board carpet covered the floor and various articles of furniture were placed in special positions, I believe Jack held the position of Tyler himself for many years after 'Tinman' Taylor died.

In the first few years of their existence, the Operatic Society held their rehearsals in the Parish Room and in my youth many privately arranged dances were held there.

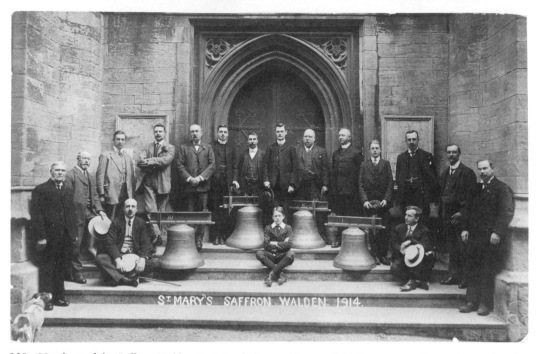

120 Members of the Saffron Walden Society of Change Ringers. This picture was taken in 1914 when four additional bells raised the peal to twelve. They were dedicated 27 June 1914. *Left to right:* Chas Freeman, J. F. Penning, R. A. Strong, A. F. James, Churchwarden John Gilling, Curate the Rev G. M. Benton, expert from the Bell Foundry to hang the Bells, Vicar the Rev J. J. Antrobus, Fredk Pitstow, Curate Rev G. F. Hart, Harold Pitstow, Alfred Pitstow, Alfred Evenett, Walter Parish. *Seated:* Fred J. Pitstow Jnr, Leonard Pitstow and Geo H. Sparrow.

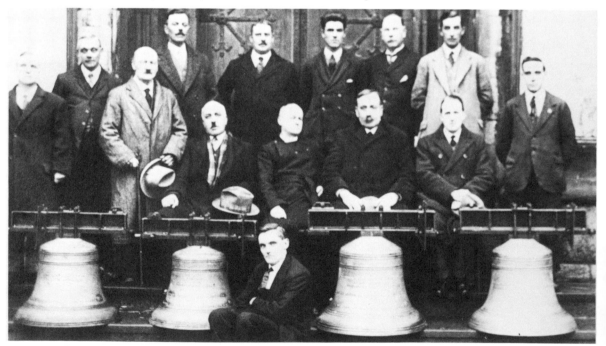

121 Dedication of four new treble bells, 15 December 1928. *Standing left to right:* G. H. Sparrow, F. H. Dench, E. A. Pitstow, Police Inspector F. Ridgwell, A. F. James, Len Simmonds, W. Parish, R. A. Strong, H. Sketchley. *Seated:* Fred Pitstow Jnr, The Vicar (Dr Hughes), Alfred E. Pitstow, Leonard Pitstow. The man in the front came from the Bell Foundry to hang the bells.

Len Pitstow is, I think, the only surviving member of the Society of Change Ringers as at that time. Mr Dench and Len Pitstow (son of Ernest) joined the Society in 1915. Between the two Wars Mr Dench, a well-known composer and conductor, rang many peals, conducting his own compositions.

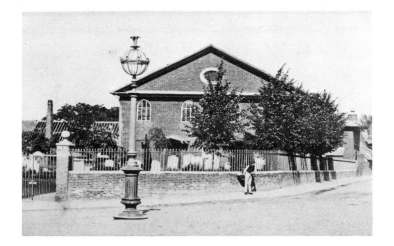

122 Baptist Church ('Upper Meeting') – built 1774. In 1760 the Rev Joseph Gwennap came to Walden and in 1764 became the Minister of the 'Independents' (now United Reformed Church) at Abbey Lane.

After worship on 12 June 1774, Gwennap was voted out of his pulpit because of differences about adult baptism. Gwennap and the majority of attenders adjourned to Sister Elizabeth Fuller's house (claimed, on strong evidence to be 'Myddylton House'). She offered her barn in Bailey's Lane (Audley Road) where worship was conducted for 21 Lord's Days. Such was the tenacity of Gwennap and his followers, that only 12 days after being turned out of Abbey Lane, the foundation stone of a new Meeting House was laid 24 June 1774, and on 6 November 1774, they worshipped in it.

The lamp-post has its own history. From about 1837 to 1863 it stood in the centre of the Market Place To make room for.the fountain, given by George Stacey Gibson and his mother to commemorate the marriage of the Prince of Wales, the future King Edward VII, the lamp was moved to the top of High Street.

After the 1914–18 War, the lamp had to make room for the War Memorial and the lamp column was moved to the pavement in front of the Ingleside Terrace houses. When the Borough Council decided to turn street lighting over from gas to electricity, I conferred with Tom Cloughton, the Borough Engineer, as to how best the old lamp column could be saved. He re-designed the top part as it is today, converted to electricity, and the Council were pleased to save this bit of old Walden. Let us hope the new people in authority today will treat the lamp-post with the respect it deserves.

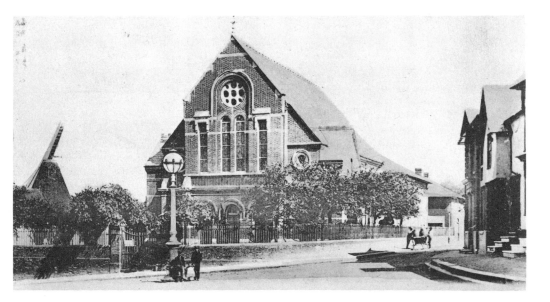

123 Baptist Church – built 1879 – photograph 1881. Pastor Rollason proposed at the centenary celebrations, that improvements should be made to the 1774 church, with the result that it was decided to build a new church on the west, or street side of the existing one, using the old building as the Sunday School and for other church activities. The work was completed in 1879. The picture of the first church just shows behind the Manse on the right-hand side, the top of the malting kiln recently demolished. This picture (postmarked 1905) shows the kiln which stood only a short distance from High Street/Gold Street corner.

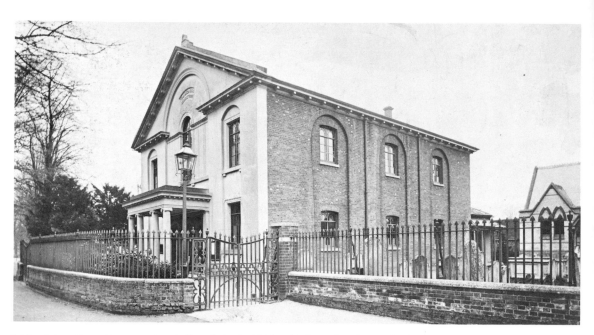

124 Abbey Lane Congregational Church built 1811. The first church was built 1694. Between 1689 and 1694, a congregation met regularly in a barn in Abbey Lane. The wall shown in the picture was built originally to the height of the railings. The railings, I believe, were removed during the 1939–45 War, when such material was required to make munitions.

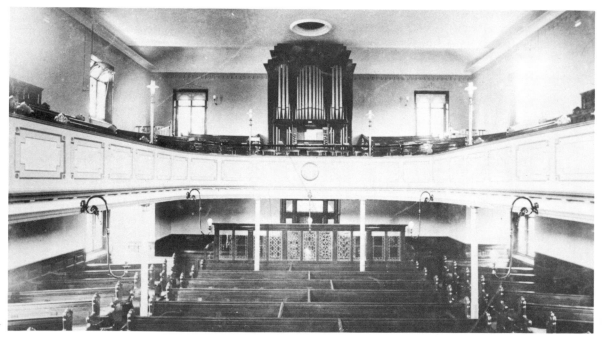

125 A view of the interior taken from the pulpit showing the organ above the church entrance.

During the ministry of the Rev George Hogben (1856–58) namely on 9 June 1858, it was decided to erect an organ in the gallery, 'where the singing pew now is, costing £160, as per plans submitted to the meeting by William Hedgeland, Organ Builder, of London'. About 8 years after the organ was erected, additions were made to it costing another £140.

At the time I write this, the organ is undergoing a thorough overhaul and repair at a cost of between £4–5,000, I believe.

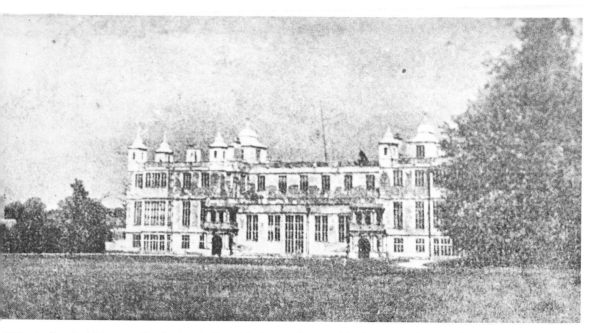

126 Audley End Mansion. South view in its original state. Engraved by Stewart and Burnet from a drawing made by J. R. Thompson from Sketches by Winstanley for the *Architectural Antiquities of Great Britain*.

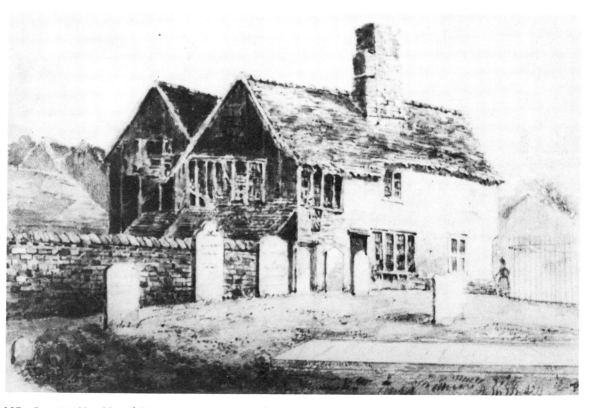

127 Opposite Nos 11 and 13 Museum Street was Thomas Bunting's house shown in the drawing by Maynard. The Bunting family were glaziers. Jonathan was a celebrated bellringer and clarinet player. The wall on the right is the end of Isaac Marking's slaughterhouse and stable premises. The wicket gate led into the churchyard.

The churchwardens bought the house from Lord Braybrooke in 1838 for £210 to demolish and provide more burial space.

Houses

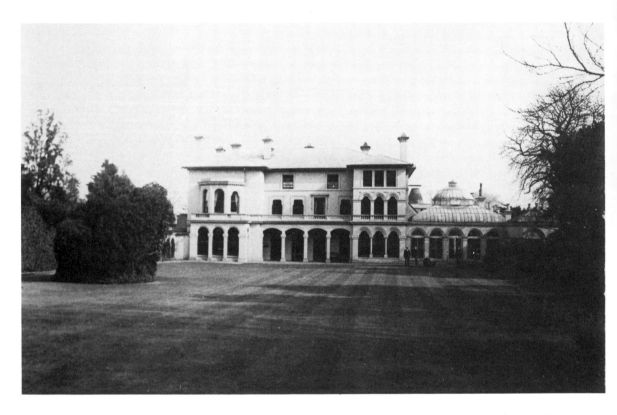

128 Hill House, High Street. One of ten pictures of the house and garden taken some time before and after February 1934, given to me by Albert Fitch not long before he died. Albert was apprenticed in the Hill House garden about 1914 under George Barker. He stayed until after Miss Gibson died 18 March 1934, when he was appointed the Borough Council's Head Gardener. He lived in the Gardener's House, No 19 Castle Street, until he retired about 1966 when he and his wife moved into a Gibson Free Dwelling in Abbey Lane.

Albert's wife was on the Hill House domestic staff so they were the last Gibson servants to occupy a Gibson Free Dwelling – almshouses built specially for retired and elderly Gibson employees. Albert died in October 1979.

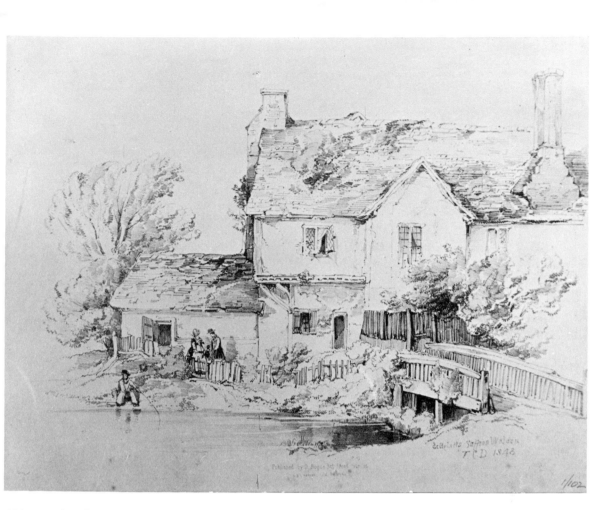

129 St Aylotts by T. C. Dibdin, 1843. Earliest authentic date for St Aylotts is 1248, Sub-Manor survival. House dates *circa* 1500.

130, 131, 132 The Close – No 2 High Street as it was from about 1854 to 1934 (*see both photographs opposite*). In the 1620 Manorial Rental, this property is described as *Priours*. It consisted of two houses the one built between 1400 and 1500, the other in 1554 which was almost entirely encased in brick by Francis Gibson in 1854. The latter part (brick building in pictures) was pulled down in 1934 and re-erected at West Grinstead for Sir Ralph Harwood, Deputy Treasurer to King George V whose hobby it was to purchase and restore old Tudor houses. In 1954 I traced the house, now called *Walden Close* and without its brick encasement, which was then occupied by the Misses Loring, who sent me a photograph of it (*see below, on this page*).

Francis Gibson married Elizabeth Pease in 1829 and lived at the Close which, in 1854, he encased with brick. His main hobby was landscape gardening and finding insufficient scope in the small Close garden, he acquired land called *Hoggscroft* behind the Castle Street houses, designed and laid out what came to be known as *Fry's Gardens*, with entrances in Castle Street and Bridge End.

Francis's daughter, Elizabeth Pease Gibson (the Gibsons perpetuated the surnames of their wives in naming their children) married Sir Lewis Fry of Bristol, a Solicitor and Member of Parliament. Francis Gibson died on 19 December 1858 and his estate eventually descended, through the daughter, to the Frys. Francis was also an artist and it was he who founded the Gibson Picture Gallery in the Castle Street entrance to the gardens. Throughout my lifetime, the gardens have been open to the public without charge.

The original *Close* garden, surrounded by a high wall, was bought by public subscription in 1936 and presented to the town. After lowering the height of the wall, erecting a shelter and laying out the garden, it was officially opened on 1 September 1938.

The Close was used as a convent up to about 1914. The large room with the gable end at the Castle Street corner was the chapel. The nuns ran a school for girls. The oval window is not now in the same position as shown in the picture. It was moved when the plaster was removed and the timbers exposed.

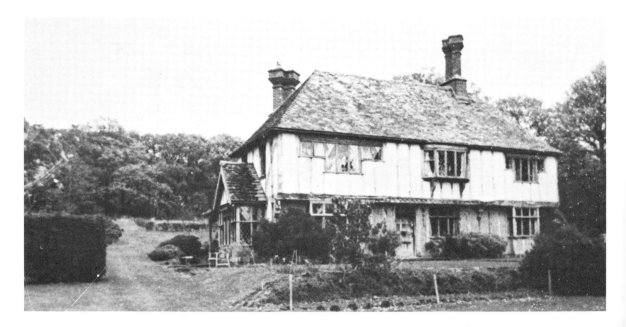

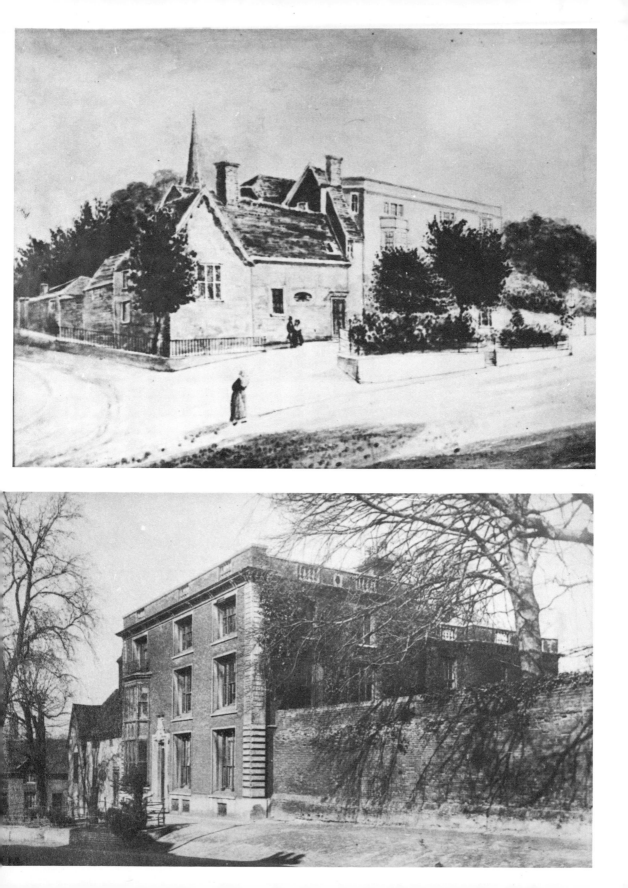

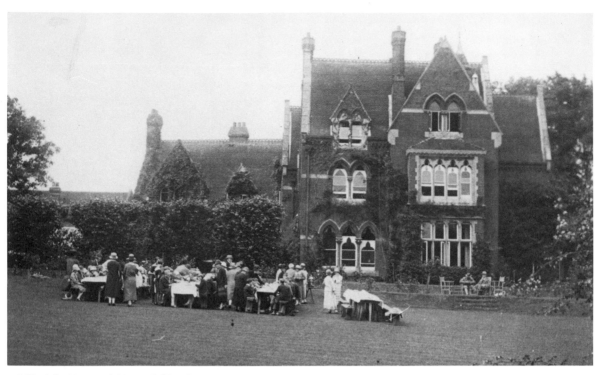

133 The Vineyard 1927. Children's tea party given by the Women's Conservative Association in the garden.

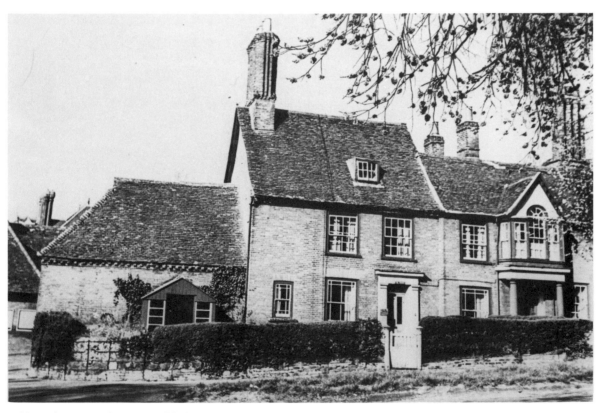

134 The Priory, Common Hill before it was altered. After Miss Elizabeth Day died in 1978, the two houses, Nos 2 and 3 Common Hill, fortunately fell into the hands of Mr Russell Hawkes the owner-occupier of No 2, and he converted the two houses into one.

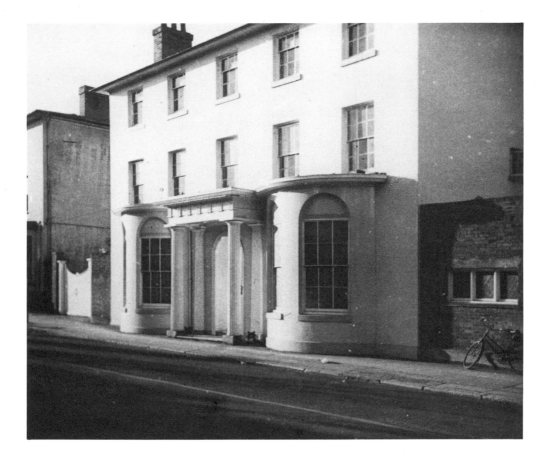

135   No 53 High Street built and occupied by Wyatt George Gibson, father of George Stacey Gibson.

Wyatt G. Gibson, born 1790, married Deborah Stacey in 1817 and lived first 'opposite his father', namely in the property now Nos 4 and 6 High Street. It was there that George Stacey Gibson was born, 1818.

Wyatt G. Gibson later built *Larchmount* in London Road and lived there for a time. Then he built 53 High Street and lived there until his death in 1862. His widow, Mrs Deborah Gibson, died 25 February 1877 aged 83. Dr Hedley C. Bartlett was living there in 1892 and he was succeeded by his son Dr Justinian Bartlett. When he retired and left the town, the property was acquired by Messrs Wild, Hewitson & Shaw, who converted the premises into a solicitors' office.

Inns

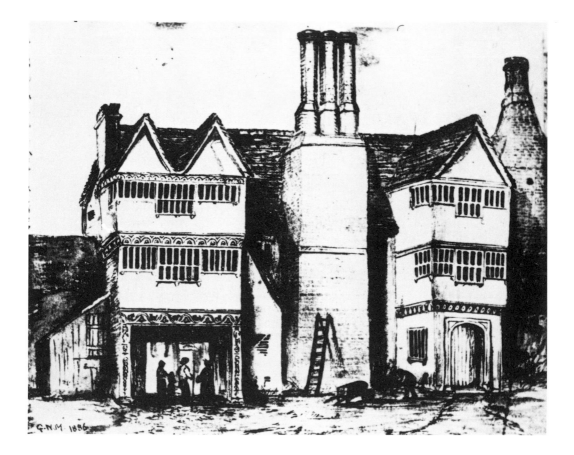

136 *THE BELL*, site of Cheffins' Cattle Market in Market Street. This is a copy of a picture in the Museum of a property which was pulled down in 1855 and the materials sold. Two stately mantels went to the Museum. One of them stands in the entrance hall. Gabriel Harvey, born in 1550, educated at Walden Grammar School, to become Doctor of Law at Oxford, a learned orator and poet at Cambridge, friend of the poet Spenser, was reputed to have lived here in the 16th century.

The Bell is mentioned in the Churchwardens Accounts for 1638. William Impey converted the inn into a dwelling-house in 1818 and the sign of *The Bell* was moved first to Cuckingstool End Street, then to 38 Castle Street which, in 1902, became the first Co-op of which my grandfather was a founder member.

Robert Paul (Mayor 1838 – died 1839) the last owner-occupier, bought three adjacent small properties which blocked up the southern exit from the Market Place into Hill Street, leaving a way only 18 feet wide between the *Black Boy* (one of the properties) and the *White Horse*.

The Council acquired the properties, demolished them and widened the road to its present width of 45 feet. Scruby's wine and spirits shop on the corner, was originally the *Town Arms* and opposite, on the site of the present Borough Market, stood the *Eight Bells* acquired by the Council in 1831.

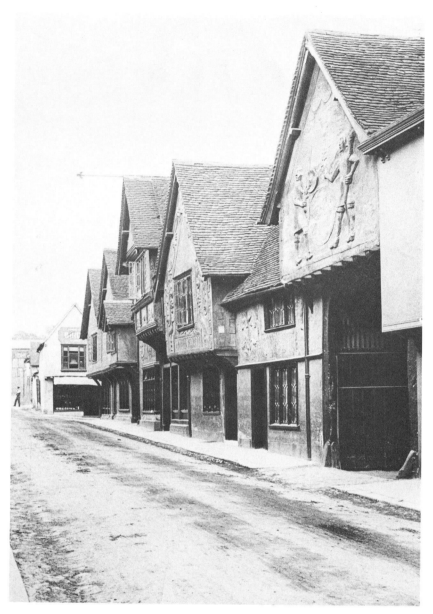

137 Church Street – *SUN INN* – *circa* 1910. Taken before Church Street was tar-macadamed and when it had cobbled gutters. F. C. Bird had his antique shop at the top of Market Hill (No 14). The man in the distance stands at the entrance to the *King's Arms* yard (see plate 141).

The gateway to the rear of the *Sun Inn* was usually left open because various people had rights of way over it. Turner Collin once owned the building at the end of the yard where his *Nats Club* had their meetings and which was later the Town Bandroom. For the last half-century or more this building has been owned and occupied by Reed & Son the antique dealers. The solicitors in Lime Tree Passage, King Street, had a right of way through to Church Street and properties in Market Hill had similar rights, I believe. Mr Cain, builder and undertaker, had his business in the yard for years.

Nos 25 and 27 were always separately let.

In the early 1930s I helped my chief, Town Clerk William Adams, with a local appeal for subscriptions enabling the property to be handed over to the National Trust. It was a Gibson property and Miss Gibson was a most generous subscriber and the G. S. Gibson Trustees made it easy for the proposal to be carried through. In the event, it could not go direct to the National Trust, but was held for it by the Ancient Buildings Trust.

138 *ROSE AND CROWN*, Market Place. A third-class passenger arriving by train, requiring to be taken anywhere in the town, hired the station bus operated by the *Rose and Crown*, seen here with Mr Osborne, who lived in Castle Street, up 'on the box'.

The bus had seats right and left, passengers being able to see out of the side windows. Steps were let down to get in and out. The luggage was carried on top.

The 'aristocrats' hired the carriage seen coming from the yard on the left, with Mr Searle on the box.

Mr Searle (who lived in Common Hill) had a son who was also employed at the *Rose and Crown*. His job was to collect and deliver from the railway station all small parcels. He had a light horse-drawn van covered with canvas. When the van was empty, or nearly so, the 'tail-board' would be left down, an invitation we could not resist to jump up at the back and have a ride, until someone shouted 'whip behind', when the long whip lash would come over the top from Searle to clear us off.

The *Rose and Crown* was burned to the ground at Christmas 1969 with the loss of eleven lives. It has now been re-placed by Boots the chemists and the only remains to be found are the bunch of grapes, now hanging from the façade of Boots, and the shell canopy over the front door which has now been set into the brickwork in the yard at the rear.

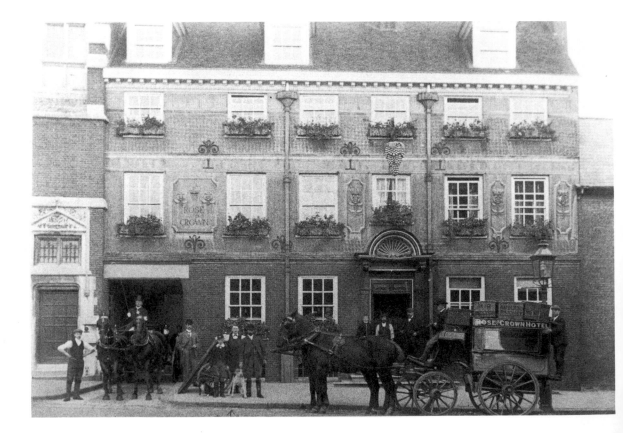

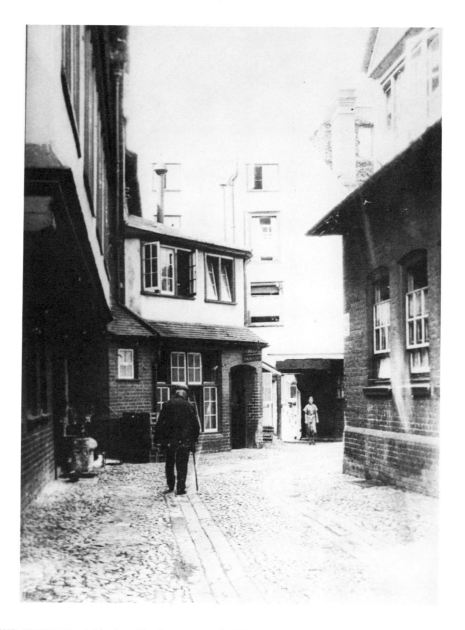

139 *ROSE AND CROWN* Yard. The hotel kitchen was on the left, the dining-room above it. The entrance to the lounge and front bar was on the left of the passage leading to the Market Square (by the girl).

The 'Tap' was the building on the right. The 'better off' drank in the 'Rose' – the lower orders 'in the Tap'.

On Market Days the cobbled yard and cart sheds would be filled with carts and traps of all kinds, the horses accommodated in the stables.

Local organisations used to have their annual dinners, followed by an entertainment, in the large dining-room.

140 High Street – *DUKE OF YORK circa* 1880. Bought by Hannibal Dunn, with land at rear, for £900 – 23 July 1845.

Note Donkey-cart on the left in front of the shop of Robert Cowell, boot and shoe maker. He was there according to the Directories covering 1887 to 1907. His daughter, a clerk in the post office, married Robert A. Strong a master at the Boys' British School.

The horse and cart outside the inn looks very much like the Royal Mail van, but it does not have the Royal markings. The window above the donkey's head displays china.

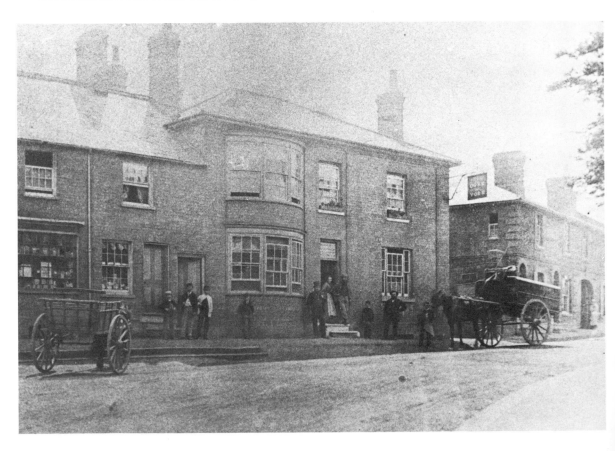

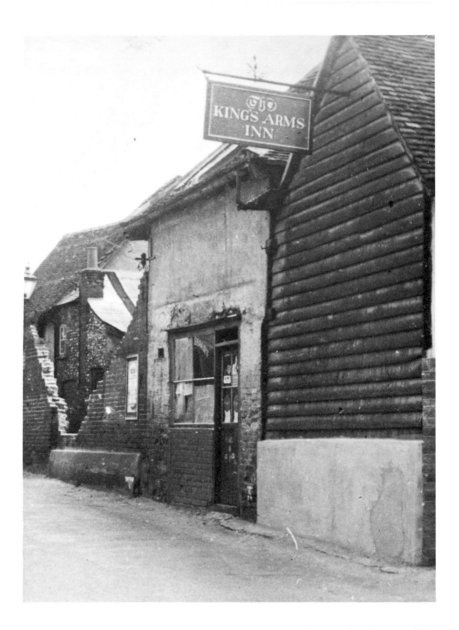

141 Church Street. South side next to the entrance to *KING'S ARMS* Yard, before demolition in 1952. The first building was Arthur Badman's cobbler's workshop.

Beyond the hole in the wall was C. Medcalf's coal merchant's yard and adjoining it, standing a little back from the road, was Davis Jeffrey's blacksmith's shop. Jeffrey lived at 16 Castle Street and his assistant, Albert G. Coe, at 25 Bridge Street. When Mr Jeffrey died, Mr Coe succeeded him in the business.

The whole site was cleared and re-developed by Messrs Cleale.

(Photo by Walter de Barr)

142 *THE HOOPS* and vicinity all decorated for the occasion of George V Coronation, 1911. In the group on the left I can recognise Albert Swan (the hatless boy left of the girl), later to become an engine driver.

The Hoops, at the corner of Cross Street (formerly Potters Row) has retained its name for over 200 years, it being first mentioned in a deed dated 1740. In 1752 *The Hoops* was described as in King's Street – evidence that *Market End Street* was renamed at least two centuries ago. The deeds relating to the property extend as far back as 1587, so one would not be surprised to find behind the modern plaster exterior the same kind of Tudor timbered building as adjoins it on the other side of Cross Street, or like the *Cross Keys* at the former *Middle Ward* end of King Street.

There is no foundation for the claim that Samuel Pepys stayed the night at *The Hoops*. Pepys stayed at *The White Hart* which manorial records of the period show stood at the corner of Church Street and High Street, namely, on the site of *Cambridge House*.

For several years the *Saffron Bloom Lodge of Oddfellows* held their meetings in the large room upstairs, now *The Old Hoops* restaurant. It was here, as a teenager, I was initiated a member of the Adult Lodge, coming up from the Juveniles. I remember knocking the door to gain admission, waiting for the spy-hole to open and a voice asking me for the password.

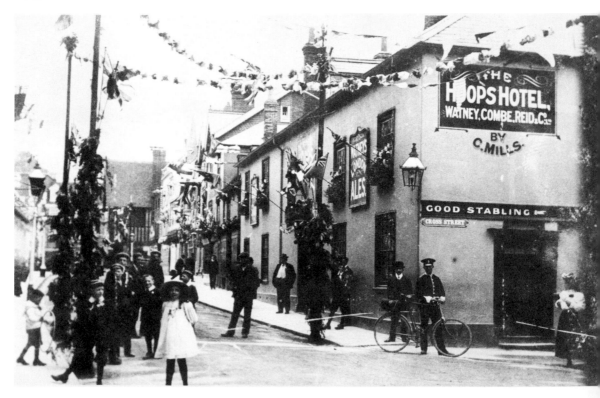

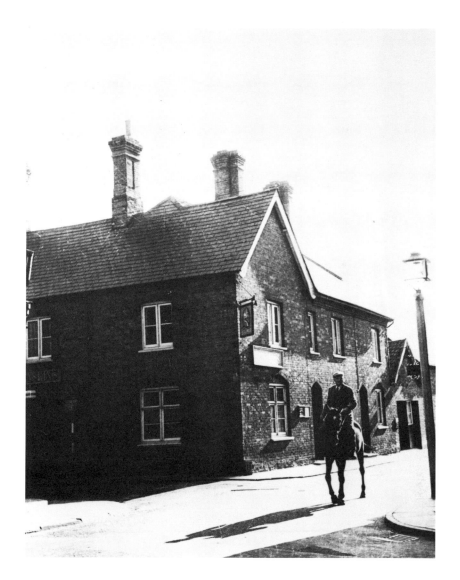

143 George Street. *THE GEORGE*, No 2 Gold Street and the George Street, No 8 entrance. No 6 was the blacksmith's house, the smithy being next to it.

As early as 1824, William Spicer occupied the public house and Richard Spicer, the smithy in *George Lane*. They were still there in 1839. By 1904 George Badman occupied the inn and engaged also in the business of a chimney sweep. His sons, Charles (Bridge Street) and William (London Road) each continued in that business. Arthur, another son, was, for years, a clerk in the Council Office. Ben, another son, was manager of the Employment Exchange where the Essex & Suffolk Insurance Office is now.

The George was a Benskins Brewery house as also was the *Greyhound* at the High Street end of George Street (see plate 144) and No 6 and the smithy No 4, also belonged to Benskins.

Planning permission was granted to F. Bell & Son for their sign (seen over the smithy door) on 23 August 1955, and for the conversion to shops, etc, of *The George*, smithy and *Greyhound* stables and yard, 19 January 1962, so this picture was taken between those two dates.

Planning permission for Budgens new shop (formerly the Co-op) was granted May 1969.

Hart's 1900 Directory records in an advertisement that W. Clark was the blacksmith 'for 5 years Manager there for Mr Hasler'. I suppose either Hubert Bell or his father was the last blacksmith to shoe a horse in George Street.

The George was one of 17 alehouses licensed in 1786.

144 *THE GREYHOUND*, High Street 1949, with Miss Muriel Pledger at the entrance.

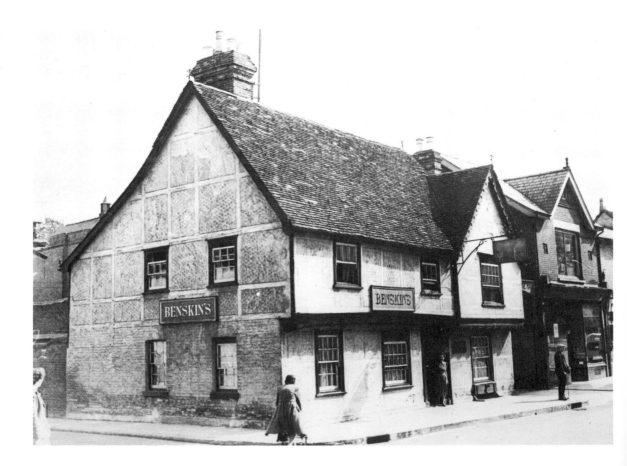

Excavations

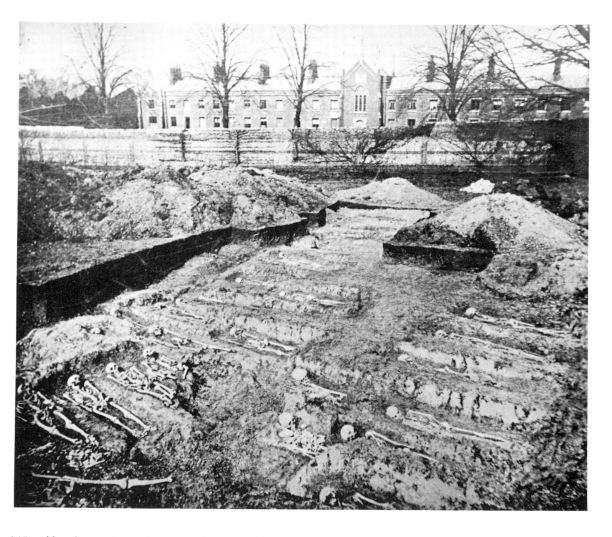

145 Abbey lane – Saxon Cemetery. Excavations by G. S. Gibson, 1876. The New Almshouses in the background locates the site. Some 150 skeletons were found where chance finds had been made in the 1830s.

Frank Emson's 1904 History of Walden, *Transactions of Essex Archaeological Society*, vol 1, part 2 (third series) in the Town Library and Report of Excavations made in Battle Ditches in 1959, page 141, can be referred to for more detailed information.

146 High Street – Gold Street Corner. Archaeological excavations undertaken in 1973 on the site of the demolished Sainsbury Malting.

The Interim Report of the Director of Excavations dated 18 August 1972, stated: 'The site, until recently that of a malthouse, is due for redevelopment for housing in the current year. Initial machine trial excavation in late December 1971, proved that landscaping immediately prior to the construction of the malthouse had entirely removed any pre-existing archaeological deposits; natural chalk was encountered directly beneath the floor screed.'

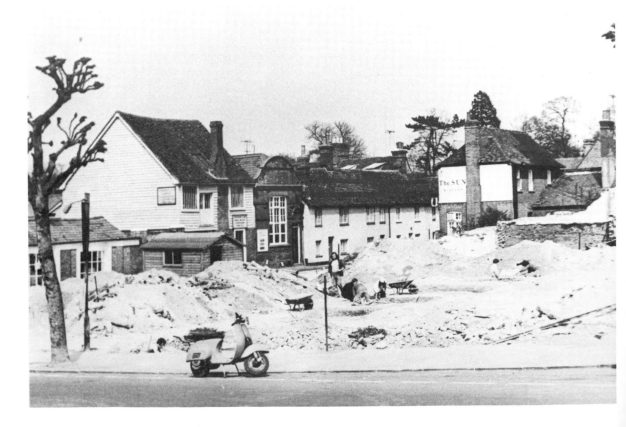

Open Spaces

Borough of Saffron Walden.

LIST OF STALLAGES AND RENTS PAYABLE AT THE FAIRS HELD WITHIN THE SAID BOROUGH.

	£	s.	d.
For every Stall at per foot frontage, per day			2
For every Caravan, Show, and Public Exhibition, Tent, or other erection for Public Amusement at per foot frontage, depth, or diameter whichever is the greater, per day			2
For every Engine drawing on the Common	2	2	0
For every Caravan, per day. . . .		2	0

No Engine will be allowed to draw across any Public Path.

The above Stallages and Rents were ordered to be leviable and taken in the said Borough at a Meeting of the Town Council of the said Borough held on the 10th day of February, 1922, and to come into operation on the 1st day of March, 1922.

W. ADAMS,
Town Clerk.

SAFFRON WALDEN,
21st February, 1922

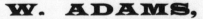

BLOOM & SON, PRINTERS, MARKET PLACE, SAFFRON WALDEN.

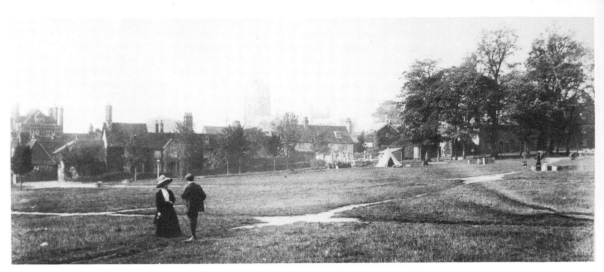

148 The Common. On 30 April 1892, Thurgood and Sons advertised in Hart's Directory their half-yearly Repository Sale on the Common. After J. Thurgood died, Mr H. J. Cheffins intended to continue the sales. His first one was a flop, mainly because of the inclement weather.

About a fortnight later, Harold Woodward arranged a sale of his own which proved a great success on a beautiful day. He continued these quarterly sales for about 25 years, until the Town Council asked for a prohibitive hiring fee for the Common which destroyed the profitability of the sales.

The picture shows the tent Mr Woodward had erected to serve as his office. Lot numbered stakes were driven into the ground in rows with ample space between for displaying farm carts, machinery, tools, harness, hurdles, stack-cloths, surplus farm equipment, etc, and allowing the auctioneer and buyers to pass up and down and do their bidding.

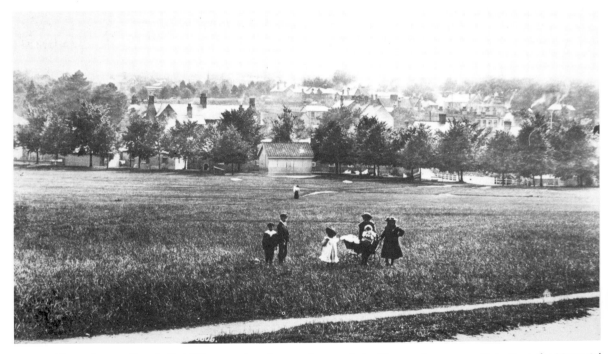

149 The cricket pavilion, built 1871, was taken down and re-erected with some improvements to it, on the Memorial Playing Field Cricket Ground, to be first used there in 1954. Before the 1914–18 War, not only was the cricket pitch it-self surrounded with bushes every close-season, but an area to the left of the pavilion was also prepared and protected as a practice area. The two white bare patches in front and wide of the pavilion were caused by schoolboys who used the trees opposite for wickets. In the summer months we used to get to school at least by 8.30 am to play rounders in front of the pavilion which was 'home'. The square formed by the two 'wicket' trees and the two bare patches was the 'rounder'. Billy *(Mop)* Whitehead usually captained one team and Alf Housden the other. The aim of course was to swipe the ball from the left-hand end of the pavilion, under the lime trees into the Slade. Happy days!

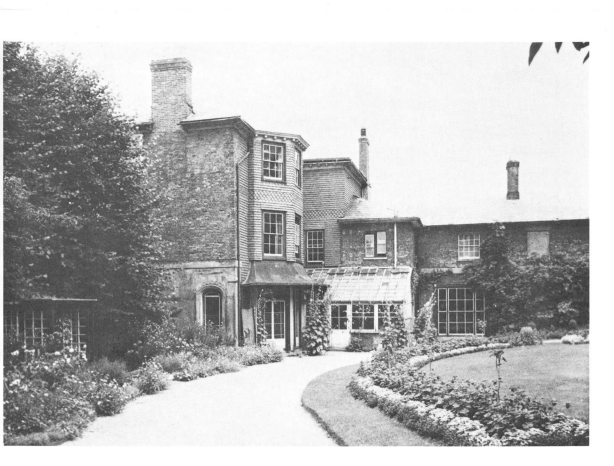

150 Jubilee Garden, Hill Street. When Town Clerk Wm Adams retired in 1935 necessitating a change in staffing, the Borough Council bought No 5 Hill Street from Mr H. J. Barrand and converted it into the Municipal Offices.

The lean-to greenhouse or conservatory was converted into an office at the beginning of the war – the first Food Office. The room to the right of it with the large window became the Committee Room. The rooms above it belonged to Cheffins. The General Office was through the glass doors under the canopy, the Town Clerk's office above it and at the top, the Borough Engineer's drawing office.

Nineteen thirty-five was the Silver Jubilee Year of King George V and Queen Mary and to commemorate the event, the garden, named 'Jubilee Garden', was given over to the town to be maintained as a public garden.

When I left Adams & Land to join the Council staff in April 1935, I worked alone in this new office for a month or so before the Council moved in from No 3.

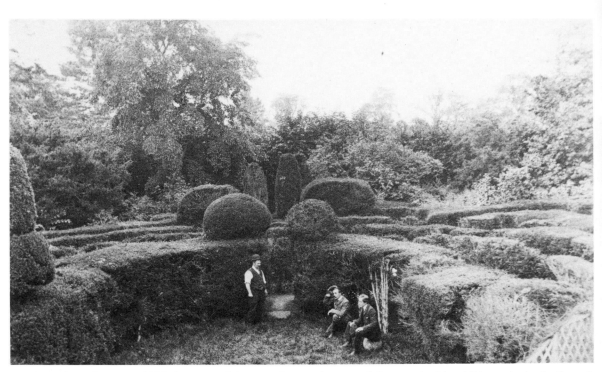

151 Fry's Gardens *circa* 1905. A picture of the maze I remember so well. It was ruined by children who broke through the yew hedges to get to the centre shown in the picture.

  This maze was a puzzle one after the style of the one at Hampton Court, entirely different from the one on the Common. I tried many times to find the middle, more often than not coming up against a dead-end and a turn round to try another way. The picture gives some idea of the winding paths to get to the middle.

  The maze was not freely open to the public. Mr Swan, the head gardener (in shirt sleeves in the picture) employed by Mr Fry, held the key, but one could pay sixpence to Mr Swan who would unlock the gate and afford entrance.

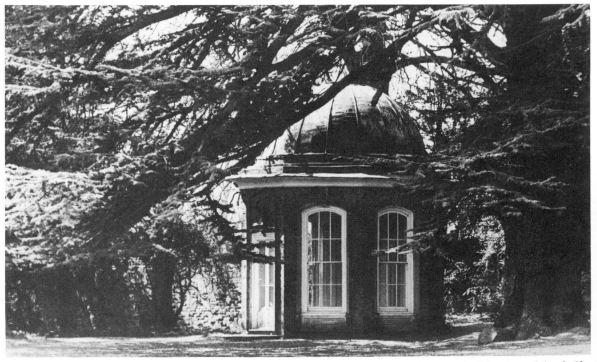

152 Summer House in Fry's Gardens. The last time I saw this lovely summer house it had been vandalised. The interior paintings on wall and ceiling were, I believe, executed by Mr Lewis Fry, father of the late Dr L. S. Fry.

Vehicles

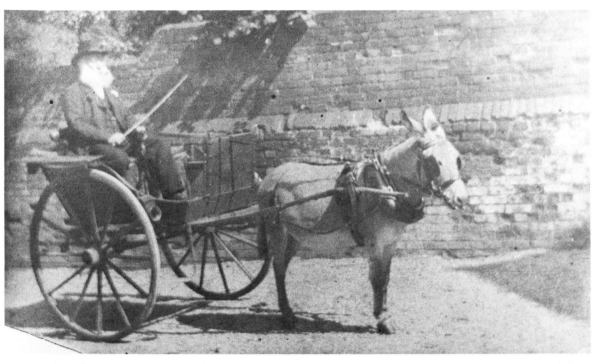

153 John Adams, 1901. Carpenter of the Shortgrove Estate, lived at 2 Bellingham's Buildings, travelled to and from work in his donkey-cart. The donkey was kept in a stable in Lower Square. John lived next to my grandfather. He was the father of George, Alec and John. A prominent member of the Oddfellows Friendly Society.

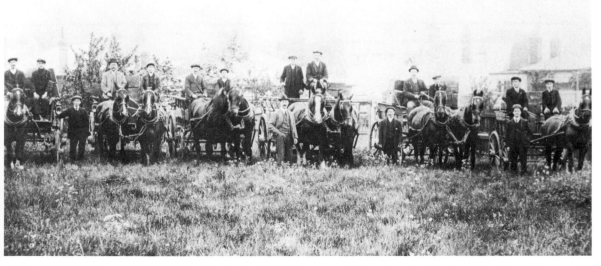

154 Staff of Robson & Co Ltd, Station Street *circa* 1913. These vans delivered goods (cleaning materials, kitchen requisites, brushes, and paraffin oil) not only to town shops, but to the villages as well. *Left to right:* Fred Start, J. Woodley, Bill Goodwin, – Freeman, *A. Bassett, Alf Archer, Peter Start, F. H. Doggett (Manager), *Frank Start, Chas Brooks, Tom Porter, Charles Pettitt, Wm Cornell, Harry Perry, Fred *(Shrab)* Bacon, Sam Harris (standing below Perry).

*Killed in 1914–18 War.

155 Newport Road, 1900. Miss M. W. Gibson's coachman Alfred Martin, (who lived near Hill House in the way to Barnards Yard and Battle Ditches) in the cutting in Newport Road before it was sloped back after World War I to provide work for the unemployed.

Newport Road was lowered in 1826 at the point where Claypits Road (which followed the course of Seven Devils Lane) crossed the London Road along the line of the hedge by Beeches Close and Sedcop Hill (by County High School) across Wenden Road, roughly to where Ice House Lodge now stands.

In 1827, the hill was lowered from Port Bridge (where Slade, by Fulfen, flows under road) to the Borough boundary at top of Sparrows End Hill. Newport Parish Council declined to co-operate with Walden Vestry on their side of the boundary. The whole of the new Gallows Hill Road, 18 feet wide, was lined with stones 6 inches deep.

These and other road improvements were undertaken to provide work for men and boys who would otherwise have had to be supported by poor relief out of the rates.

Fred Mallion, a local man, returned to civilian life soon after the 1914–18 War, having served his time in the Regular Army. He was employed as a charge-hand with the gang employed sloping the cutting referred to above. There was a fatal accident during that work, a great quantity of chalk falling on and burying one of the workmen. Fred Mallion proved his worth on that contract and stayed with the Borough Council to succeed George Goodwin as road foreman.

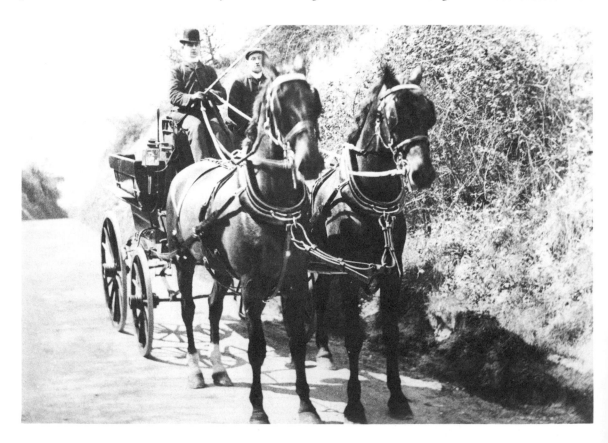

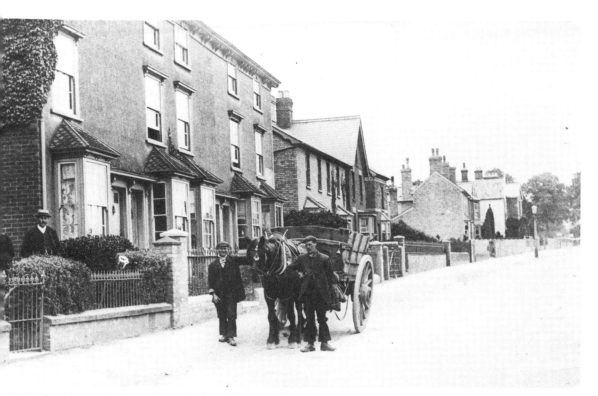

156 The Corporation Dust-Cart collecting refuse in Radwinter Road about 1912. *Note* the bell hanging in front of the cart to warn householders that the collection was being made.

157 The Borough Council's Steam Roller outside Miss Earnshaw's house, 85 High Street and Sid Golding's sweet-shop at corner to Battle Ditches and Barnards Yard on right of it. *Left to right:* 1 A. Archer; 2 ?; 3 Jim Smith. Who can name No 2 for me please?

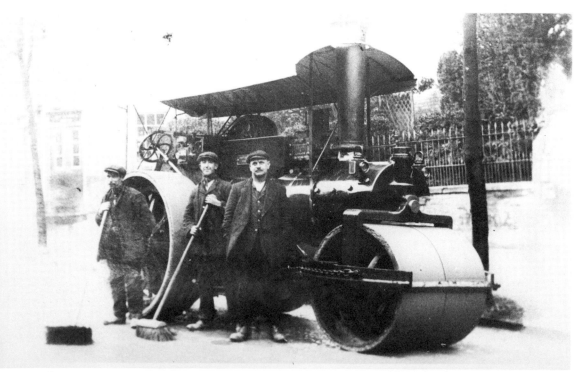

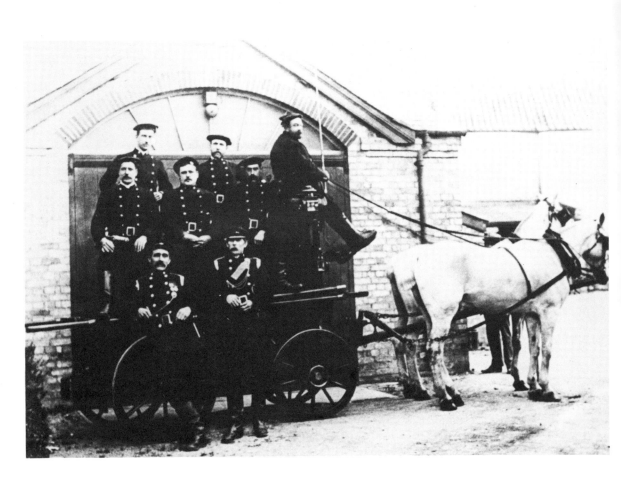

158 This photograph would have been taken between 1905, the year Arthur Day joined the Fire Brigade, and 1907, the year Dick Williams resigned. All seven firemen were later to be awarded Long Service Medals, an outstanding record of public service. *Back:* E. H. Cro (1900–26), J. B. Burton (1896–1920). *Centre:* A. E. Whitehead (1902–26), A. Day (1905–27), Albert Housden (1903–26). *On ground:* George Wyatt (1896–27 – Foreman 1904–20 – 2nd Officer 1920–27), Andrew Robert Dix (1889–1920 – Captain 1903–20), Driver R. A. Williams (who supplied the horses from his livery stables in Freshwell Street) 1900–07.

At this time the Fire Brigade had to be called out by pressing a bell in a recess made in the front wall of the original Council Officess, No 3 Hill Street, next to the Fire Station. Members were not individually connected with any alarm system. The bell, which connected with the Police Station, was behind a glass panel which had to be broken before pressing the bell-push. The police did the 'calling-out'. At some stage the siren at the Gas Works called the men out. Before telephones became the common means of communication, there was inevitable delay in getting to a fire.

This picture was taken in the yard next 3 Hill Street which was the Highways Depot and stables. The Water Softening House was on the right. The building at the back of the group was actually the Fire Engine House. When Dick Williams received the fire alarm he had to get the pair of horses out of the stable and run them from Freshwell Street to Hill Street before harnessing and securing them to the engine. Here again valuable time was lost in getting to a fire.

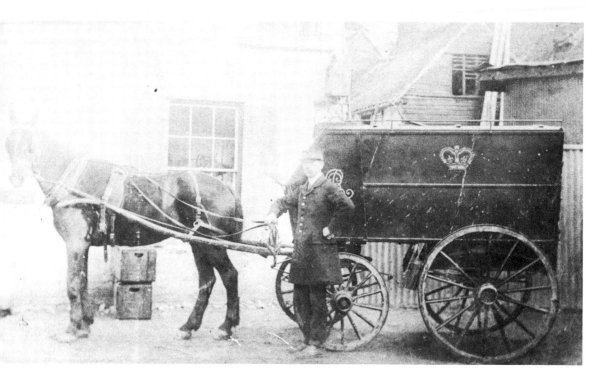

159 Mail Van with driver Jack Butcher. No 9 Church Street was the driver's rest and harness rooms, harness on ground floor, a bed upstairs. For many years now No 9 has been occupied with No 11. The door of No 9 has been blocked up.

In between mail collections at Audley End Station and any other port of call, horse and van were kept in the yard between Nos 7 and 9. The stable and cartshed for the van were in the yard through the gates. The provision of a horse, a driver, stabling facilities, etc, was a job the Post Office contracted out and if my memory is right, Arthur Titchmarsh had it. The driver had awkward hours and had to get his rest as he could.

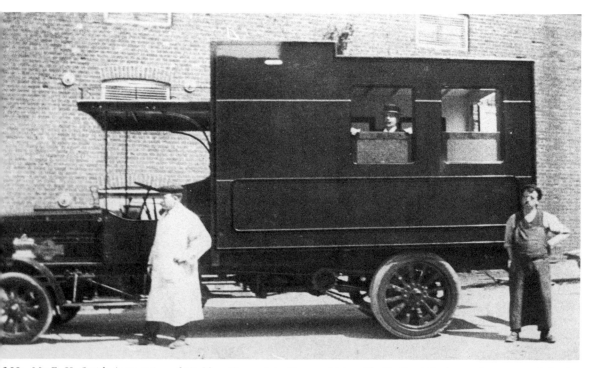

160 Mr E. H. Smith (proprietor of Walden Cinema) inside a vehicle with Mr Fred Taylor at the rear end, in the Maltings Yard below the Cinema (High Street). The driver of the van is unknown to me.

161 Joseph Wright outside his shop Nos 26–28 High Street (now Woolworths) *circa* 1904. I was told that the car outside belonged to Lord Howard de Walden when he was at Audley End Mansion.

In 1907 Mr Wright was agent for Humbers, Rovers, Singers, Swifts and Gladiators and advertised '300 Cycles always in stock to select from. Prices to suit all from £5 new. Tel No 016.'

In 1914 he was sole agent for Humber, Belsize, Daimler, Darracq, Arrol-Johnson, Swift, Austin, Rover, Sunbeam, Flanders, BSA, Unic, Hupmobile and Crossley. Tyre stockists for Dunlop, Michelin, Continental, Wood-Milne, Mackintosh.

His son, Frank P. Wright, also advertised in 1914 as Authorised Sole Agent for Saffron Walden and District for *Ford the Universal Car* and agent for Swift, Humberette and Singer Cycle Cars and any other make.

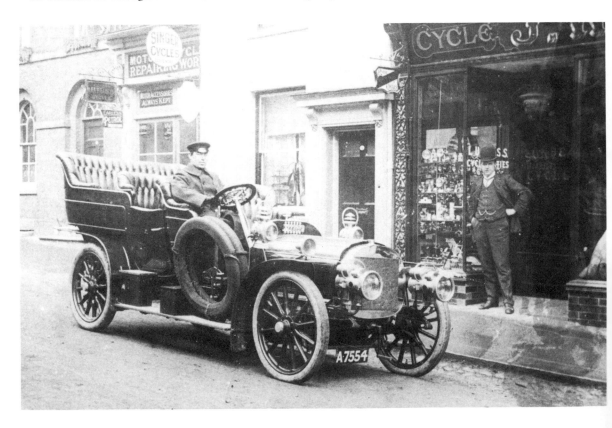

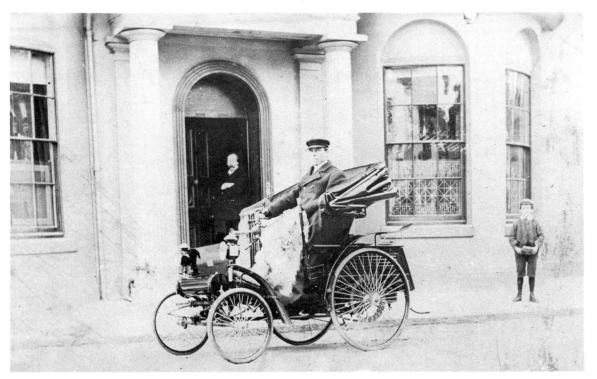

162 Dr Hedley Coward Bartlett at his front door of 53 High Street and his waiting car, an early Benz, said to have been the first in Walden. The driver is Walter Green, a former groom. In 1904, Doctors Bartlett and Bascombe were in practice together.

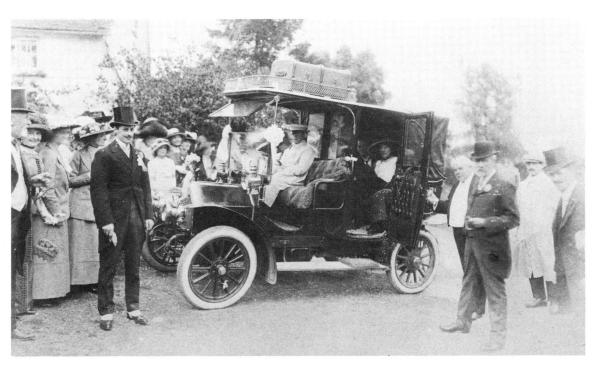

163 I discovered this picture under another I was taking from its frame. It is interesting as showing an early type of car.

The first man on left is Henry Myhill who farmed Dawkins Farm, Hempstead and retired to live in Ivy Cottage, London Road, Saffron Walden. On extreme right is Charles Nott, who married Henry Myhill's daughter Amy, sister of Mrs K. Holland (widow of George Holland) who lived at the Old Mill, Wenden.

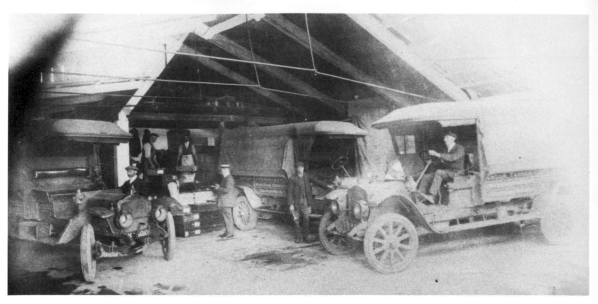

164 One of the Motor Garages at Emson & Tanner. *Left to right:* Harry Notley, George Underwood, John Cowell, Charles Coe, Jack Mumford with Manager John Green wearing a straw hat in centre.

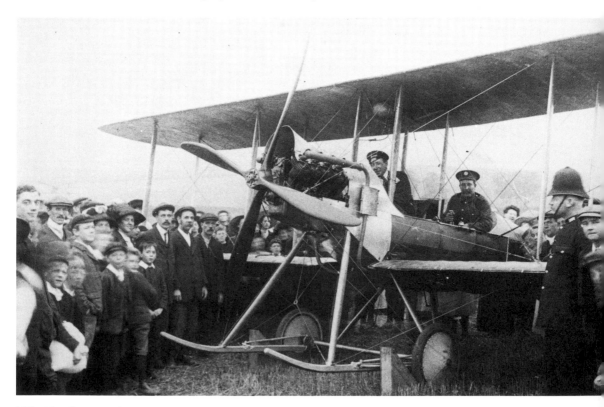

165 This flying machine came down about 8.30 one morning in the autumn of 1912 during army manœuvres in this part of the country. It landed first near Shire Hill Farm, but took off to hop over Thaxted Road to the large field beyond Coe's farm in Peaslands Road.

The town turned out to see this wonder – a biplane actually on the ground! Frank Wright (son of Joe who had his motor salesroom where Woolworths is now in High Street) has told me the pilot came down in Walden because he wanted some engine repair done. On a previous occasion (at Littlebury I think it was) Frank had done a similar job for him.

When we got to school we were given the morning off so that we could go and see this new invention.

Various people in the picture are still living.

Special Occasions

166   London Road *circa* 1862/63. Five of these pictures were given to me by Miss Stokes and Mrs Sims who worked for Miss Tuke and I was told they were taken in 1862 to commemorate Queen Victoria's Silver Jubilee.

Wyatt Geo Gibson (father of Geo Stacey Gibson) married Deborah Stacey and lived first at Nos 4–6 High Street where G.S.G. was born. Then he built the house before which this decorated structure stands on the left of it. Over the hedge on the right was built about 1864, the General Hospital, which was able to receive its first patient in 1866.

At the time this picture was taken Wyatt Geo Gibson would have gone to the other house he built for himself namely No 53 High Street at the corner of Abbey Lane (Dr Bartlett's for many years). The London Road house came to be occupied by Arthur Midgley, a grandson of Jabez Gibson, which property was called 'Larchmount'. When the 'Larchmount' garden was developed for residential purposes, it was named 'Little Larchmount'.

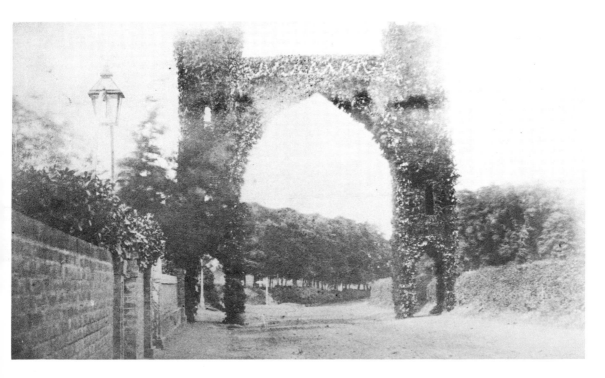

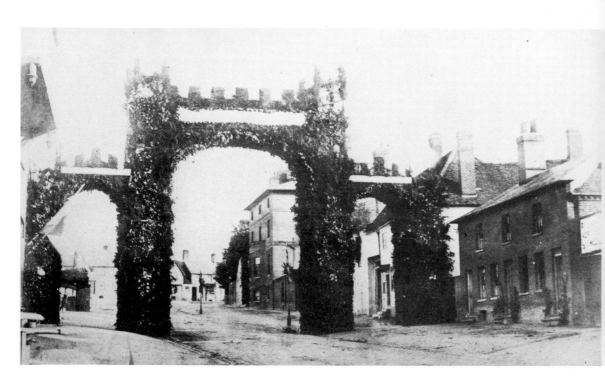

167 High Street *circa* 1862/63. A similar structure to that shown previously for the same celebration. *Note:* That Hill House had not yet been extended on its north side. That No 73 is hidden from view behind the high right-hand side of the centre arch. The three cottages on the right, behind which was the first Meeting House of the Society of Friends. In 1879 the cottages were demolished when George Stacey Gibson built and presented a new Meeting House linked to the old one.

168 The Common – Queen Victoria's Golden Jubilee, 21 July 1887. The saplings, protected by guards, are the two rows of limes along the top of Slade. The lines of bare earth are little landslides in the bank of the Slade. The people are surrounding the cricket pitch where the sports were held. Records speak of a greasy pole so perhaps the scaffold-pole erection on the right of the picture helped support it.

In the background of the picture is a high chimney which I conclude was in Copt Hall Buildings, just off Ashdon Road on the north side. These buildings comprised 20 tenements forming a terrace of 10 back-to-back houses, sideways to the road, erected with only a 4½ inches division wall. They were built in 1822 for silk weavers. In 1887 a disastrous fire occurred and 17 families were burnt out.

Silk manufacture flourished in Walden about this time. The factory went to Halstead but for what purpose was such a high chimney required?

As the Mayor, Joseph Bell, had accepted an invitation to be at Westminster Abbey on Tuesday the 21st, the Corporation attended a Divine Service in the Parish Church on Monday the 20th, afterwards going to the Common at 1.30 pm to unveil the fountain erected there. The side of the fountain records the planting of 169 trees to commemorate the Jubilee.

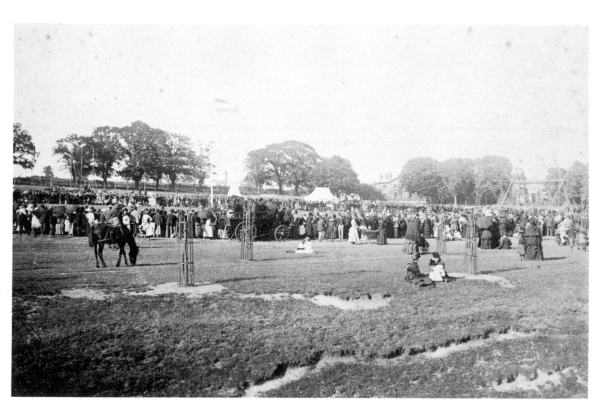

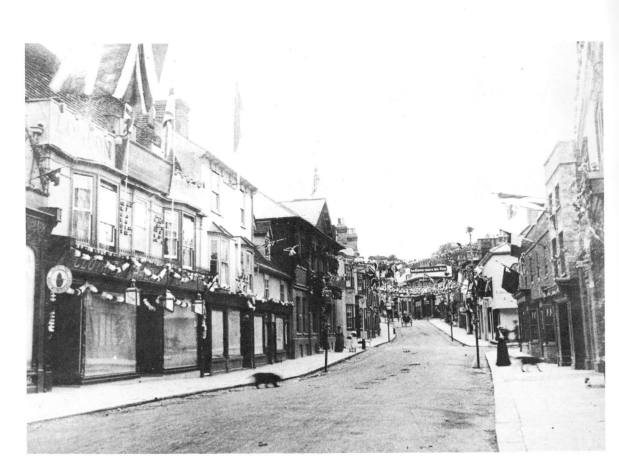

169 High Street – Coronation Celebrations, June 1902. This picture, which can be dated, shows the *London House* of Gray Palmer.

The first shop on the left was run by Geo J. Freestone, a cycle engineer and agent. Later he moved his business to 4 Gold Street. He was the son, I believe, of George Freestone the engineer and machinist of South Road.

The large house which will be recognised as today's post office, was the home and surgery of Dr J. P. Atkinson Senior.

The shop, No 41, adjoining the Atkinson house was, in 1902, occupied by the Misses Hart for their *Berlin Wool Repository*. Miss Hart later moved to Church Street.

Ernest Street, who had come to Walden from Littleport some time before 1892, had his draper's business at No 43. Mr Street was the grandfather of Sir Henry Marking and Frank, his brother.

No 45 was the home of Sidney Pidduck, later to be the home of Fred Pitstow Jnr, agent for the Essex & Suffolk Insurance Co and secretary of the Oddfellows Friendly Society.

It will be noted that the timbers of the *Cross Keys* at the King Street corner, had not yet been exposed nor the sign board moved to its present position.

At the King Street corner, George Beard had his draper's shop at Nos 34 and 36.

Walter R. Richardson, tailor and hatter, was at No 38. On the south side of No 38 was a yard over the high wall next the street. This yard, years later, became Central Arcade.

170 Coronation of King Edward VII and Queen Alexandra, 1902. The Town Band are gathered to the right of the fountain in Market Place. The men in the two ranks wearing helmets, facing the Town Hall, are not policemen, but the Volunteers of the time. I remember my father, who was a member, had such a hat. The spike was made to screw in the top. The Volunteers, like the band, are *at ease*, as if they are waiting for *the platform* to appear.

The shop, next to the London and County Bank, was occupied at this time by John Gilling, but there are notices in each window *This shop to let*, no doubt preparatory to the move of this business to Market Hill (now Chinese restaurant).

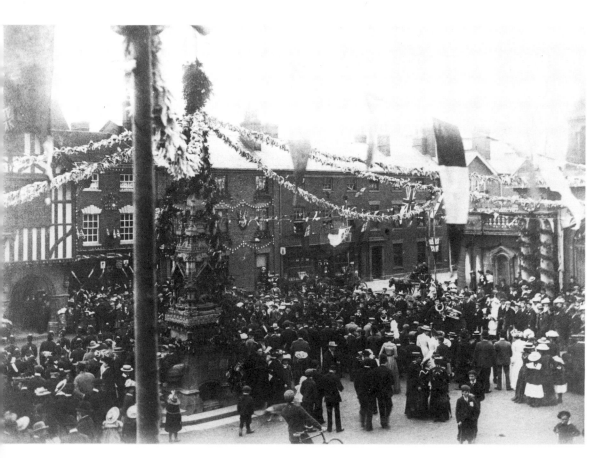

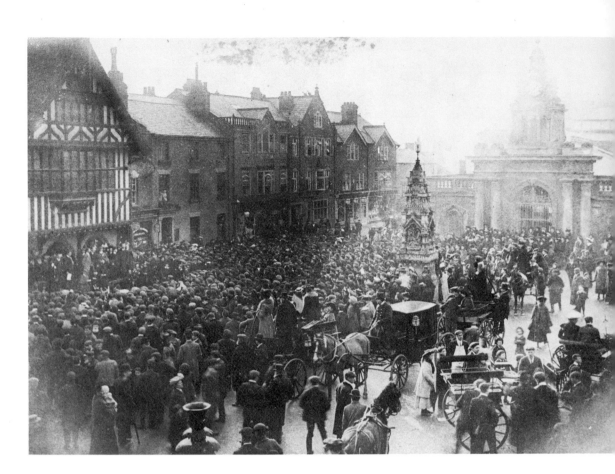

171 Market Place Declaration of Poll, 1906, 1.35 pm. J. A. Pease (Liberal) 4,203; – Bartelot (Conservative) 2,935.

Note the private carriages. Mr Pease became Postmaster-General, I believe, and was created a Baron, taking the title of Lord Gainford.

172 Empire Day, 24 May 1908. The School to the left of the fountain is the Museum Street Infants'. Mrs George Archer, Headmistress, stands next the fountain. The front row is headed by Cliff Welch and next to him is Cliff Stacey, waving his Union Jack, determined that Britons never shall be slaves!

Fred Pitstow stands on the form to conduct the singing. His brother Ernest, is conducting the Town Band which includes from left to right: Charlie *(Rufus)* Mallion; Henry Housden; Frank Champ; W. Lovell (double bass); Fred Housden in Grammar School cap in front of Lovell; Tom Marshall; ? Alf Walls; Arthur Martin.

My cousin, Glayds Housden, is the girl with the frilly hat standing back in the centre of Bandsmen Walls and Martin, close to teacher Miss Etty Smith.

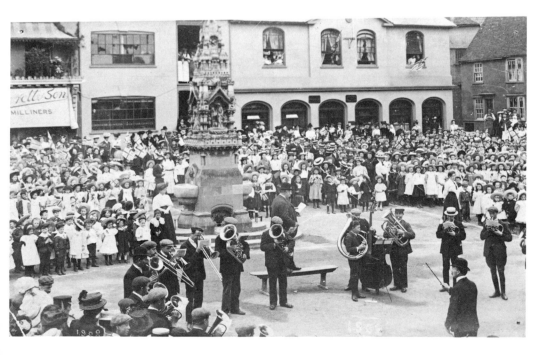

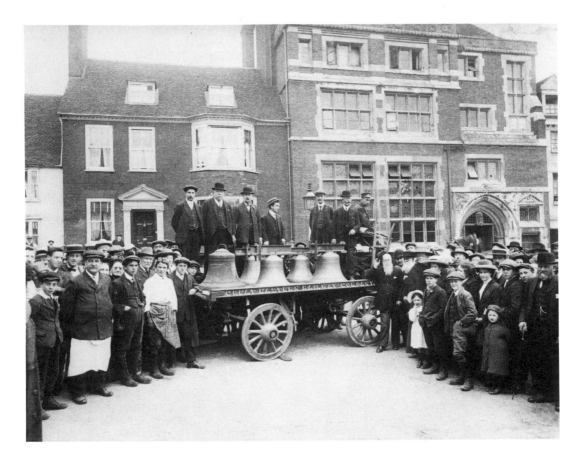

173 Great Eastern Railway van delivers the four new bells to be hung in the church belfry to make up a peal of twelve. The bells were hung and dedicated 27 June 1914.

On the van, left to right, are – man from bell foundry, Fred Pitstow, John Gilling (churchwarden), G. H. Sparrow, Alfred Evenett, J. F. Penning, driver Swan or Chipperfield. Below the driver are J. W. Burningham (holding hat), George Moss Taylor (with beard). The boy in front next the little girl is *Midget* Swan and next him George Moore. On the left are Ernie Page, Edgar Miller, Harold White, Walter Evenett, Bert Salmon, Leslie Law, Charlie King, Frank Ketteridge and Henry Housden at the back. The fifth bell (the one on the left) was being returned after making good a defect.

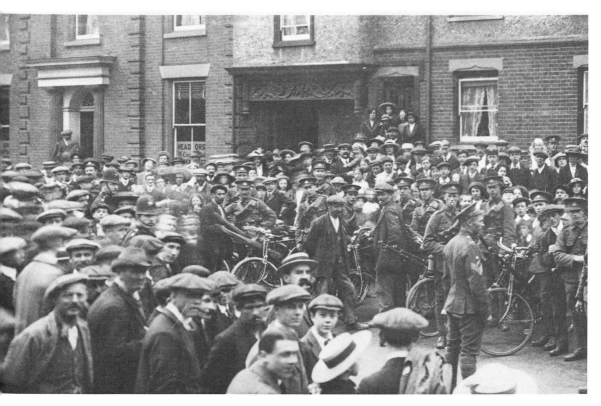

174 Departure of the Territorials (Cyclists Co) at the outbreak of the 1914–18 War, from their Headquarters, No 86 High Street. Sergeant Herberg, Ted King, Holmes from Alpha Place, – Butcher, ? W. Clarke (postman), Frank King (by wall, top right corner) are some I can recognise.

The hatless youth (between downpipe and window of No 88) is Arthur Grimes, one of the first scholars of the Boys' British School to die of wounds. Len Pitstow, Dick Selves Snr, Tommy Snow, H. M. Gillett, are among the onlookers. Fred Pitstow by window right side edge.

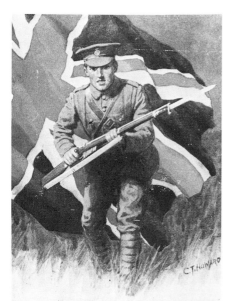

Don't be Alarmed! **We're on guard at SAFFRON WALDEN.**

175 A 1914–18 War patriotic postcard much used to keep up morale. This one bears a 1915 postmark and is in colour.

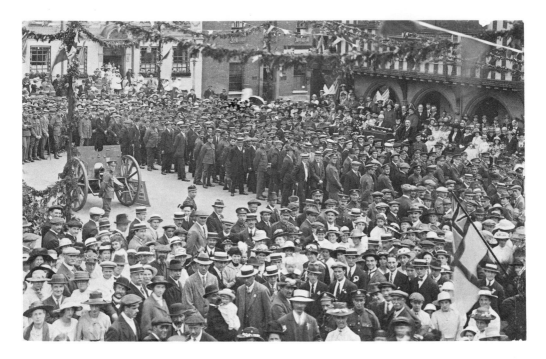

176   Peace Celebrations 26 July 1919. The field gun is one captured from the Germans and presented to Saffron Walden.

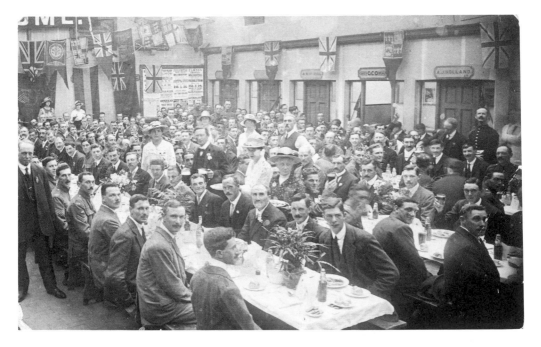

177   The returned servicemen entertained to dinner in the Corn Exchange.

178 The United States Third Air Force Band playing on the Market Square, 13 August 1955.

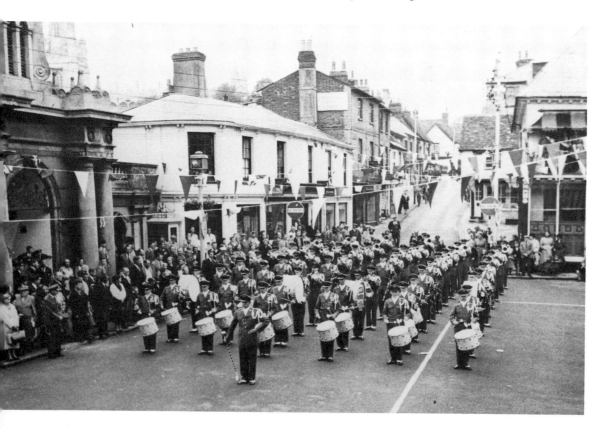

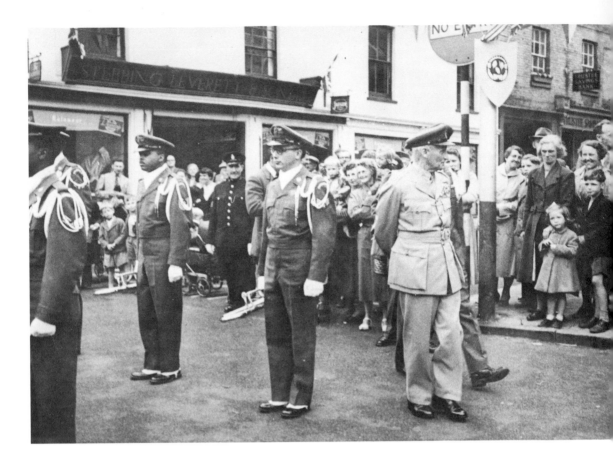

179 Anglo-American Memorial Playing Field officially opened 13 August 1955. Field-Marshall the Viscount Montgomery of Alamein, KG, GCB, DSO, inspecting the United States Third Air Force Band on the Market Place. The band, the pride of the US Air Force, came to Walden with Major-General Roscoe C. Wilson, Commander, Third United States Air Force, for the official opening of the Memorial Playing Field and the dedication of the memorial apse.

The weather was fine in the morning when the band played on the Market Place and during the official luncheon in the Town Hall, but it poured with rain all the afternoon. 'Monty' insisted that the choirboys in their surplices and no coats, sang from the shelter of the apse.

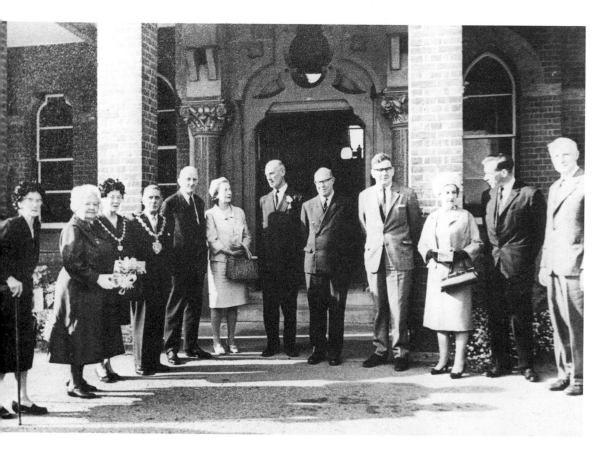

80 Hospital Centenary year, 1966. *Left to right:* Dowager Lady Braybrooke, Matron Gratwick, Mayoress Mrs Barnard, Mayor Geoffrey T. Barnard, Sir Stephen Lycett Green, Lady Green, Colonel Sir John Ruggles Brise (Lord Lieutenant), J. F. Burnet, Peter Kirk, MP, Mrs J. M. Leonard, C. H. A. Roberts (Secretary), A. L. Godfrey.

Personalities

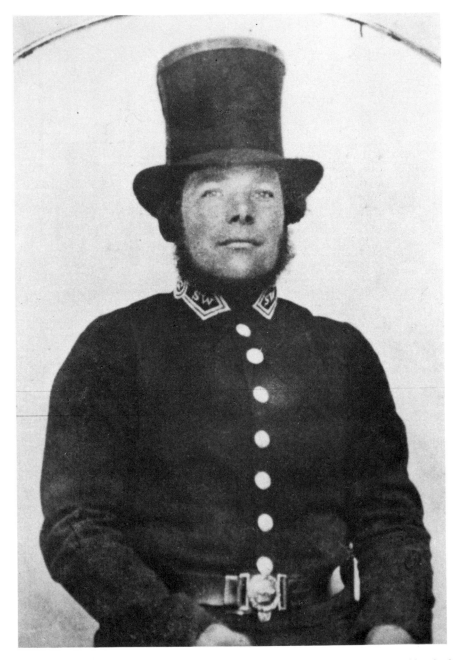

181 Thomas Duberry (or Dewberry) Constable (son of James). Before 1857 Walden had its own Police Force with a Chief Constable and two assistants. For certain special occasions, eg, Fairs, Special Constables were engaged and paid a shilling for the job.

The resignation of the Chief Constable in 1856 and the difficulty encountered in filling the post, led to the amalgamation, in 1857, of the Borough and County Police.

On 31 October 1849, Walden's Chief Constable, William Campling, was shot in the legs when he left the *Eight Bells* to cross Bridge Street to his house opposite, at 10.10 pm. Campling died of his wounds. The person charged with the murder at Chelmsford Quarter Sessions was found 'not guilty', the prosecution evidence being too circumstantial to permit of any other verdict.

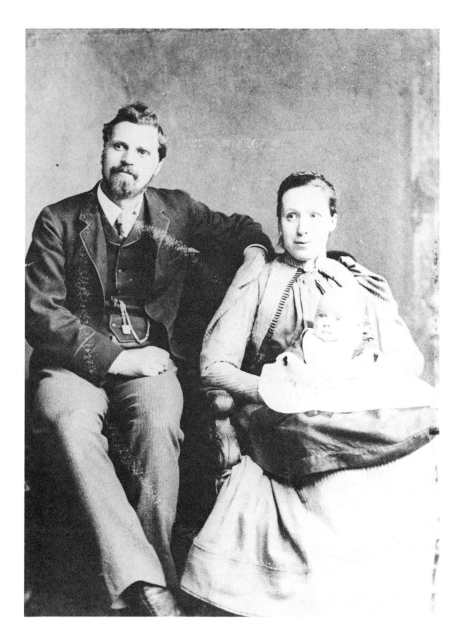

182   Mr and Mrs Wm Ernest Hart and Daughter Marjorie – 1893. Ernest was the son of Wm Hart and grandson of Henry who, in 1836, commenced business as a printer, bookseller, etc, at 21 King Street, moving later to 18 King Street (see plate 89). Mrs Mary E. Hart died 8 August 1915 aged 52. Mr Hart died 28 June 1930. Ernest was elected a Councillor 2 November 1917 and an Alderman 8 June 1928.

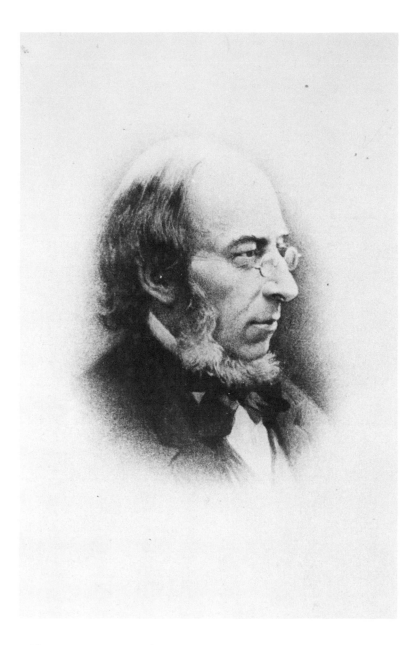

183 George Stacey Gibson. Born 1818 in High Street (now Nos 4 and 6) opposite his grandfather's house (now No 7). He was the son of Wyatt George and Deborah Gibson. G. S. Gibson married Elizabeth Tuke in 1845 and lived at 'Hill House', a property built by Henry Archer in 1821. G. S. Gibson enlarged it, particularly on the north side, and made the extensive and lovely garden. He lived there until his death in 1883. His widow died in 1890. There was only one child – Mary Wyatt Gibson born 19 April 1855, who died 18 March 1934, aged 79, a spinster.

184 George Housden, porter at the General Hospital. He lived at No 6 Mount Pleasant Cottages. He was succeeded, I believe, by Mr – Smith, and then John Adams, whose daughter, Jean, served on the nursing staff for several years.

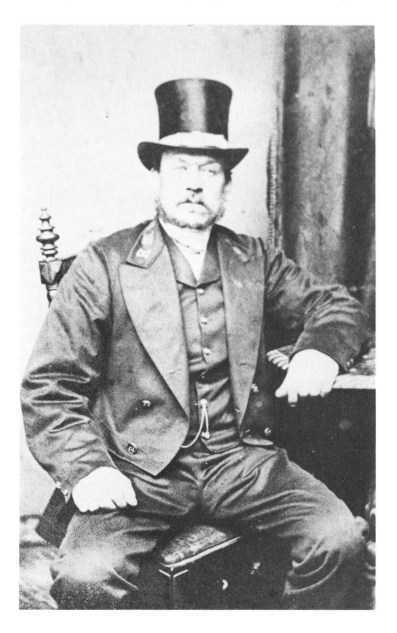

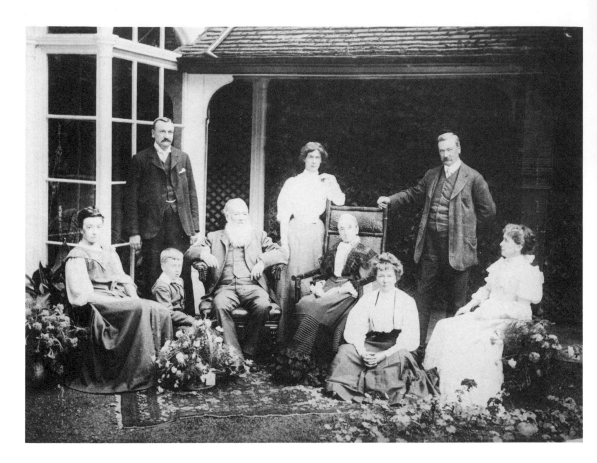

185   Alderman and Mrs Joseph Bell with family at Dorset House on their Golden Wedding Day, 1906. *Standing at back:* Arthur Bell, Miss Phyllis Bell (married Alfred Nockolds), Wm Charles Genge Bell. *Front:* Miss Edith Bell, L'Argent Bell (son of W. C. G. Bell), Mr Joseph Bell, Mrs Bell, Miss Lucy Bell, Mrs W. C. G. Bell.

Joseph Bell, a builder, was elected a Councillor 1 November 1873 and an Alderman on 10 June 1892. He was Mayor ten times, in 1877, '78, '85, '86, '98, '99, 1906, '07, '08 and '09. He died 30 December 1911, the last person to own and occupy the house as a private family residence.

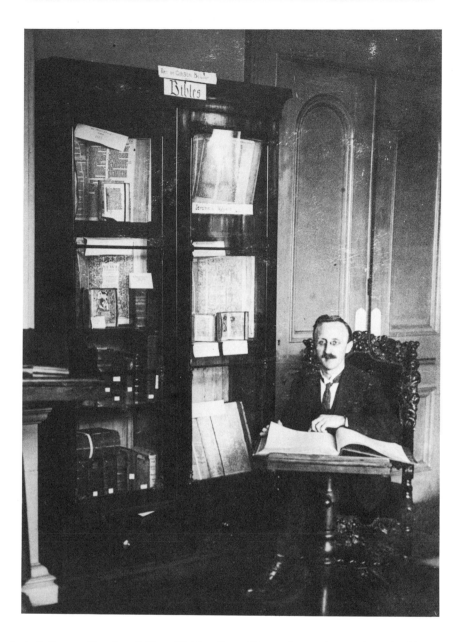

186 Arthur Ezekeil Gower, librarian, Saffron Walden Town Library (or, as it was then, the Literary and Scientific Institution). He sits before the bookcase of Bibles, part of a Gibson Bequest of 1922.

When Gower's successor failed to return to his wife and family after a fortnight's holiday, it was discovered that a number of the most valuable books in the library had gone. The police recovered some through booksellers, but the majority were lost. The absconded librarian was never found, so the police were unable to execute the warrant for the man's arrest.

187 Mr Charles Brightwen Rowntree, BA, Headmaster of the Friends' School, with his wife Gertrude (*née* Tawell). Born in Sunderland 29 October 1873, 'C.B.R.' as he was respectfully known to his intimate friends, was educated at Ackworth, Sheffield Royal Grammar School and Bootham. He left school in 1890 to become a schoolteacher. He came to Walden in 1901 to commence 33 years' association with the Friends' School, first as Senior Master and then (from 1922) as Headmaster. He retired in 1934.

Elected a Borough Councillor in 1932, an Alderman in 1949, he served as Mayor from 10 November 1947 to 26 May 1950. He was Chairman of the Housing Committee 1936–41, 1946–47 and 1950–55. It was typical of the man that when he was elected Mayor to be *ex-officio* a member of all Committees, he vacated the Chair of the Housing Committee during his term of office to allow another member to be appointed. He was re-elected to the Committee in 1950. During the war, he was Chairman of the Evacuation Committee and Food Control Committee. He served on other local committees and for a time was Chairman of the General Hospital.

As a young man, during the time he was on the staff at Sidcot School (1892–95), he played football for the Somerset Schools XI *v* Somerset County and came to Walden with the reputation of an accomplished player. By 1906 C.B.R. was playing for the Walden FC and acting as its Hon Secretary. In 1951 he published *Saffron Walden Then and Now*. C.B.R. died on 3 March 1955, aged 81 years.

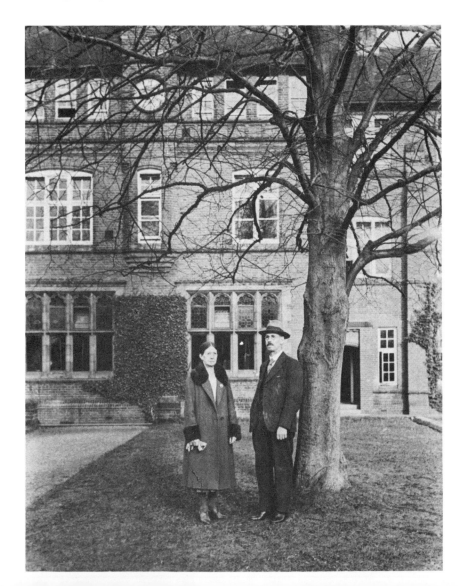

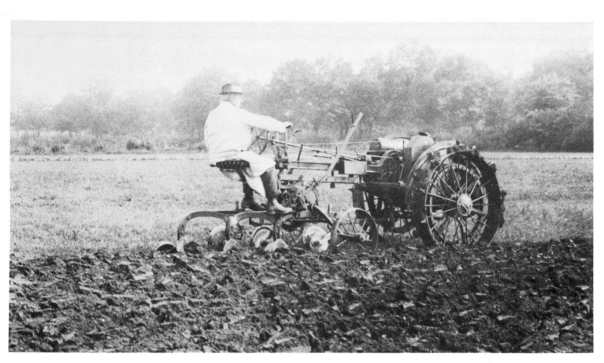

188 Councillor Arthur Titchmarsh ploughing a field in Little Walden Road, August 1917.

189 Stanley Wilson speaking to a thin audience in Market Square 1929, from a *Daily Herald* touring van, presumably to publicise the new Labour 'daily'.

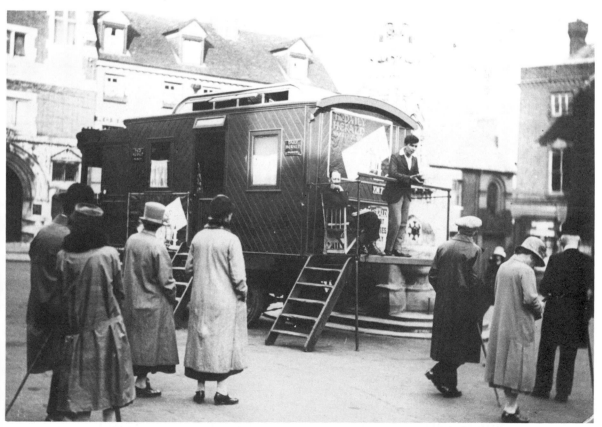

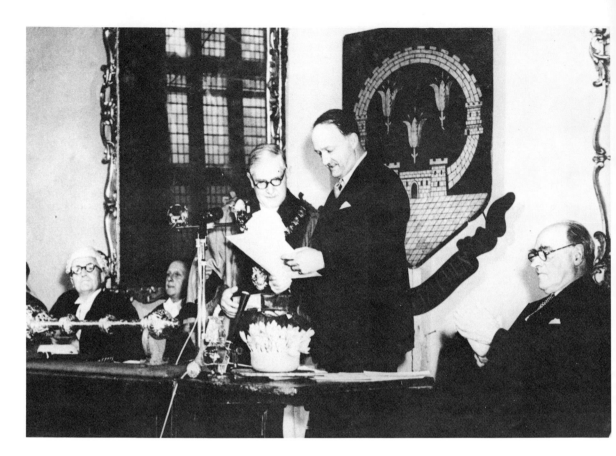

190 Presentation of the Honorary Freedom of the Borough to the Rt Hon Richard Austen Butler, CH. MP, 10 September 1954.

The Mayor (Councillor Fred Goddard) called upon the Town Clerk to read the resolution passed unanimously at a Special Meeting of the Town Council held 27 July 1954, which was in these terms: 'That this Council do confer the Honorary Freedom of the Borough upon The Rt Hon Richard Austen Butler, Companion of Honour, in recognition of the twenty-five years he has represented the Saffron Walden Division as Member of Parliament, and of his eminent services to the Nation during that time in various Departments of State, and as the present Chancellor of the Exchequer.

'That by conferring on him the highest honour it is in their power to grant, this Council acknowledges the never-failing interest which Mr Butler has shown in the welfare of the Borough, and the willing help he has given to his constituents throughout his representation of this Division in Parliament.'

After a Motion that the Honorary Freedom 'be now presented' was declared carried, Mr Butler took the Oath – '. . . that I will faith and truth bear to Our Sovereign Lady the Queen, her heirs and successors and truly to my power will maintain the Franchises of the Borough of Saffron Walden and truly by my power will keep the peace.'

After Mr Butler signed the Freeman's Roll, the Mayor presented him with the Certificate of Freedom together with a silver casket.

This picture shows Mr Butler receiving the Illuminated Address. The Lord High Chancellor (Lord Simonds) on right, congratulated the new Freeman, as also did Mr Recorder Connolly Gage. The bowl of flowers on the table were presented as 'Saffrons' from which Walden derived its prefix name 'Saffron'. The flowers, however, were not *Crocus sativus* but *Colchicums*, an entirely different species, but commonly called Autumn Crocus or Autumn Saffron or Naked Lady because the flower blooms in the autumn without leaves, which then appear in spring without flowers. The flower and leaves of a *Crocus sativus* come together in late autumn.

Mayor and Corporation

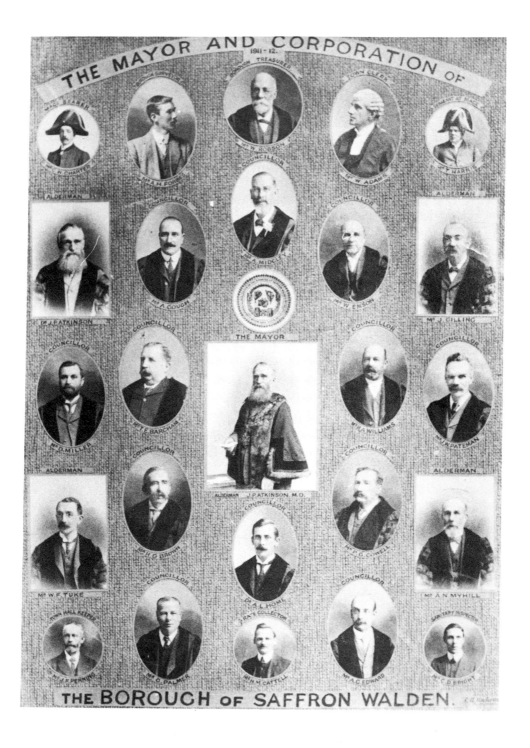

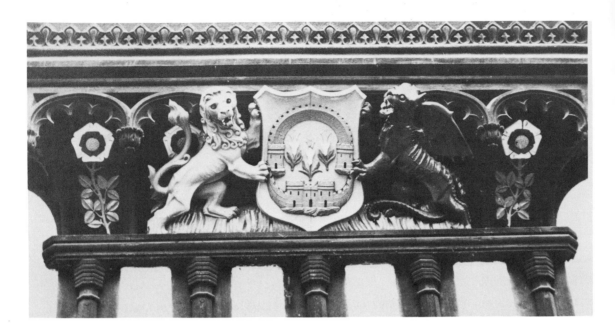

192 Borough Arms on the front of the Town Hall. Upon the stem or shaft of the silver-gilt mace of 1685, the Borough Seal is reproduced in semi-armorial fashion with heraldic supporters – a dragon on the dexter (left) side and a lion on the sinister (right) side. By the 1685 Charter, James II appointed Sir Edward Turner as first Mayor and Christopher Monck, Duke of Albemarle, as Recorder. The Duke had as supporters of his Arms, a dragon and a lion, sometimes shown dexter and sinister respectively, as engraved on the mace, and sometimes sinister and dexter respectively. An authority on Borough Arms comments 'This fact seems to be the explanation of the introduction of these animals as supporters – though it must be confessed that it was an unwarrantable heraldic liberty to have so employed them'.

It will be noticed that the supporters of the Arms on the Town Hall have the lion dexter and the dragon sinister – in reverse to the design on the mace.

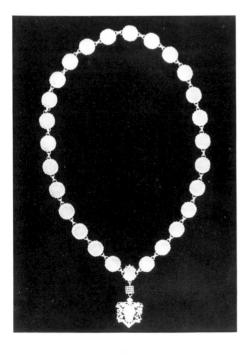

193 Mayoress's Gold Chain. This gold chain was presented in 1937 by The Rt Hon Richard Austen Butler, Member of Parliament for the Saffron Walden Constituency 1929–64. The weight of the chain is 9.55 ozs troy.

The 'office' of Mayoress is 'unknown to the law'. It is a courtesy title for the Mayor's wife or other lady acting in that capacity.

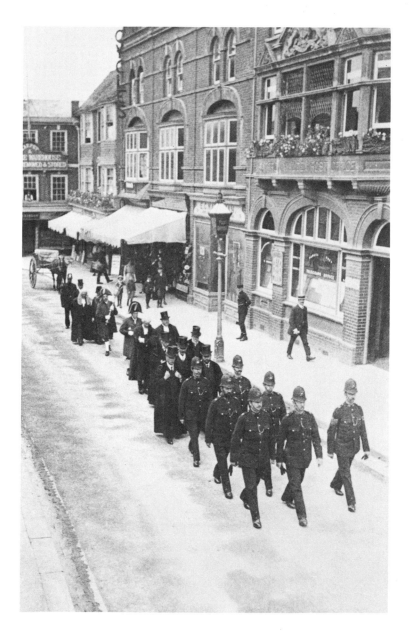

194 King Street *circa* 1913. A Mayoral procession returning via King Street from church to a Borough Quarter Sessions. Sergeant Brown and police escort followed by: E. W. Tanner, David Miller, J. W. Pateman, H. G. Brown, Addy Nunn Myhill, Wm Adams (Town Clerk), J. A. S. Baily (Clerk to Justices), Tom Harris (Serjeant-at-Mace), C. W. Charter (Mace Bearer), Recorder C. E. Jones, Mayor (Dr J. P. Atkinson Snr), Superintendent J. E. Boyce is at the end of the procession.

If the person walking behind the Mayor and Recorder is Mr C. S. D. Wade the Clerk of the Peace, then he should not be there. Only the Lord-Lieutenant, or a Deputy Lord-Lieutenant, specially appointed to represent his superior as the representative of the Crown, would have had precedence over the Mayor.

The telegraph boy outside the post office is Percy Pettitt and I think the man is Arthur James.

Charter, the Mace Bearer, resigned in 1913, E. W. Tanner had been re-elected in 1912 (November), so the picture must have been taken in the straw-hat weather of 1913.

195 The Saffron Walden Borough Council in the robes they wore prior to members being supplied with new ones in 1924. Previously members had to buy their own robes. *Standing high at back, left to right:* Borough Surveyor A. H. Forbes; Councillors E. Rooke, M. Medcalf and E. W. Tanner. *Standing, centre:* A. C. Marsh, (Serjeant-at-Mace); Councillors A. T. Greenslade, J. Custerson, W. E. Hart, A. Titchmarsh, Captain A. W. Lloyd, E. W. Hatton, E. W. Trew, JP, Dr J. H. Swanton, C. W. Rolfe, JP, Fred Sewell (Mace Bearer). *Seated:* J. S. W. Leverett (Borough Treasurer), Aldermen R. A. Williams, JP, David Miller, JP (Mayor), Wm Adams (Town Clerk), J. W. Pateman and P. G. Cowell. (Councillors Custerson and Swanton were unable to be present when the photograph was taken. The photographer used his art, took separate pictures of them and added them in the group picture in the positions they are.)

I was not undertaking Council work in 1924, but my impression is that Mayor Miller discovered that there were some forgotten funds at the bank standing to the credit of the Council – surplus subscriptions to local efforts, which the Council were satisfied they could utilise in providing new robes.

As one would expect, Councillors robes and top hats, being expensive to buy, tended to pass around when members either retired or were defeated at the polls. The old robes were infinitely better than the new ones.

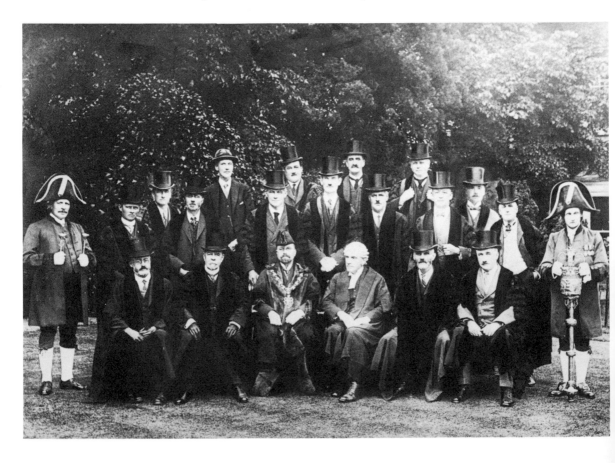

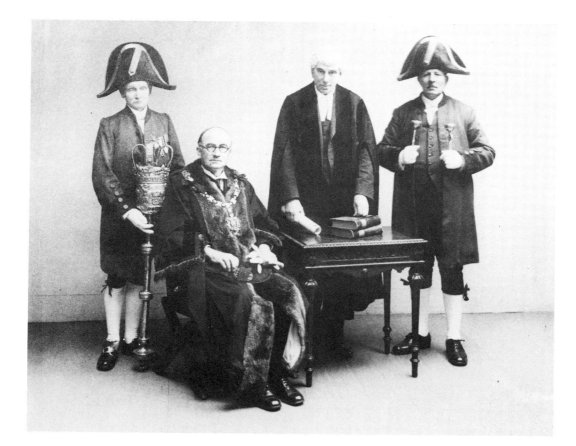

196 1 Frederick Sewell, Mace Bearer 1921–35; Serjeant-at-Mace 1935–c1945.

2 Joseph Custerson, elected Councillor 1 November 1921; elected Mayor 1931, 1932, 1933, 1944, 1945; elected Alderman 14 July 1933; resigned 4 February 1958; died 25 May 1958.

3 William Adams, DL, Town Clerk – appointed 11 April 1895; retired on superannuation 1935.

4 Arthur Charles Marsh, Mace Bearer 12 September 1913; Serjeant-at-Mace 13 May 1921; resigned 1935.

197 Mayor's Day, 9 November 1942. I believe Stanley Wilson's Churching of the Mayor procession, was the last time both Serjeant-at-Mace (Fred Sewell) and Mace Bearer (Bill Dennis) attended.

George Moore was on war service with the police and Bill Dennis, a member of the Council's building staff was undertaking George's job as Town Hall Keeper and Mace Bearer.

The uniform was in a bad state before Marsh retired and could not be replaced in wartime, so the carrying of the two small 1549 silver maces was discontinued.

Note the sand-bagging of the Town Hall, an air raid precaution measure to prevent bomb-blast effect.

The bunch of grapes customarily hanging over the entrance to the *Rose and Crown* was removed for the duration of the war for reasons of safety.

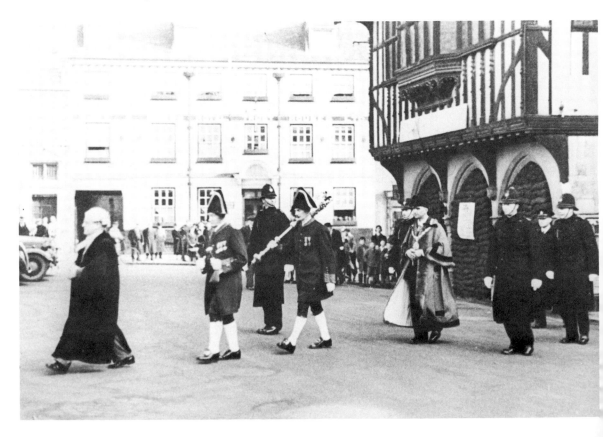

198 6 January 1951 – The Mayor (Councillor Fred Goddard) conducts in mayoral procession to the Town Hall, the newly appointed Recorder (Connolly Hugh Gage, MP, KC,) for his first Sitting of Quarter Sessions.

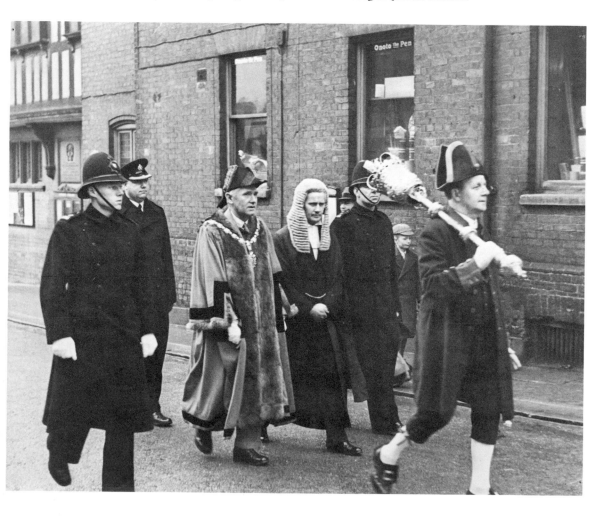

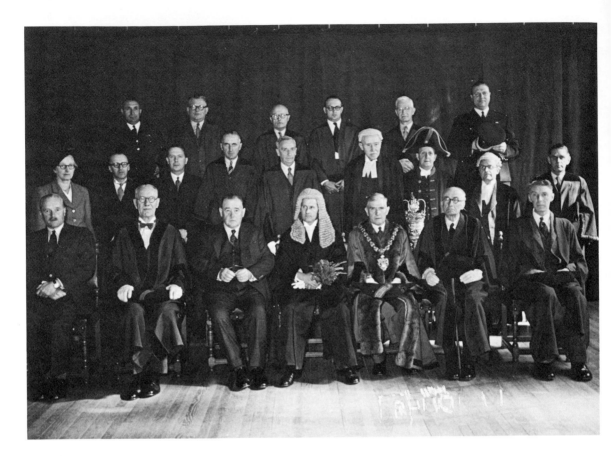

199 Last Sitting of Borough Quarter Sessions – 29 September 1951. In December 1949, Mr R. A. Butler supported an Opposition amendment of the Justices of the Peace Bill, allowing discretion of the Lord Chancellor to retain a separate Commission of the Peace of Quarter Sessions in a Borough where such a course was desirable for geographical or historical reasons, or to secure the better administration of justice.

Mr Butler said Saffron Walden, one of the oldest boroughs in the country, was threatened under the Bill 'They are frightened not only that their Recorder will be taken away, but that this is the beginning of a process which will in the end result in the borough itself being destroyed as well' he explained. 'This eating-in process is very much feared by my constituents.'

Mr Butler's fight for the Borough was not to be successful but how abundantly true his words proved to be on the 1 April 1974 when the third oldest borough in the County of Essex was reduced in status to that of a mere Parish Council.

Mr Recorder Connolly Gage is shown in the picture holding the traditional herbs. In days of indifferent water supplies, no baths, primitive toilets, no easy water heating, in fact the absence of all those facilities necessary to promote cleanliness and personal hygiene, odours in overcrowded courtrooms were unpleasant to say the least. For relief, a Judge provided himself with a bunch of herbs to smell when the atmosphere became overpowering.

When Mr Linton Thorp, KC. was appointed Recorder in 1932, he asked that this tradition be kept alive in Walden and it was the Mayor who usually made himself responsible for bringing to Quarter Sessions a bunch of herbs for the Recorder and it was my job to remind the Mayor. The herbs were usually handed to the Recorder by the Mayor in the Council Chamber before the Mayor and Corporation escorted the Recorder in procession from the rear door of the Town Hall round to the Market Place entrance.

Back row – left to right: Inspector Joslin, Cllr Fred Start, Cllr Basil E. Chapman, Cllr J. W. Barr, Cllr Arnold S. Brereton, Superintendent Simpson. *Middle row:* Mrs M. Slater, E. F. Watson (Clerk to Justices), W. J. Piper (County Clerk of Peace), Cllr Ken Foote, Cllr P. L. Allen, C. Parry Williams (Clerk of the Peace for Borough), George Moore (Mace Bearer), H. C. Stacey (Town Clerk), Cllr G. T. Barnard. *Front row:* Captain F. J. Peel (Chief Constable of Essex), Ald G. O. Bradley, Ald Ellis Rooke (Chairman of Borough Bench), Mr Connolly Gage, KC (Recorder), Cllr F. W. Goddard (Mayor), Ald Jos Custerson, Cllr A. L. Godfrey.

Groups

200 Occupants of the Gibson Free Dwellings in Abbey Lane. As Miss Mary Wyatt Gibson is in the picture with her companion, Miss Turner, I would guess that the old people were being entertained, perhaps to afternoon tea, at Hill House, which would account for the surroundings. Unfortunately, I do not have the date of the picture, nor the names of all the company. *Standing:* Miss – Smith (Miss Gibson's staff – later to be Mrs Woolnough); Mrs Lagden; ?; Miss – Pitstow; Miss Turner; Mrs Travis; ?. *Seated:* ?; Mrs Edwards; ex-PC Woodcock; ?; ?; Miss Gibson; ?; ?; Mrs Woodcock.

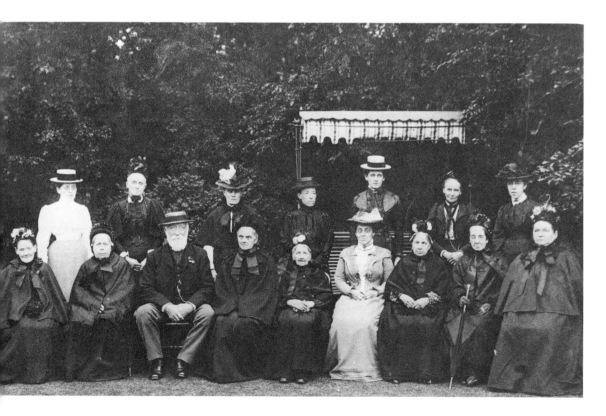

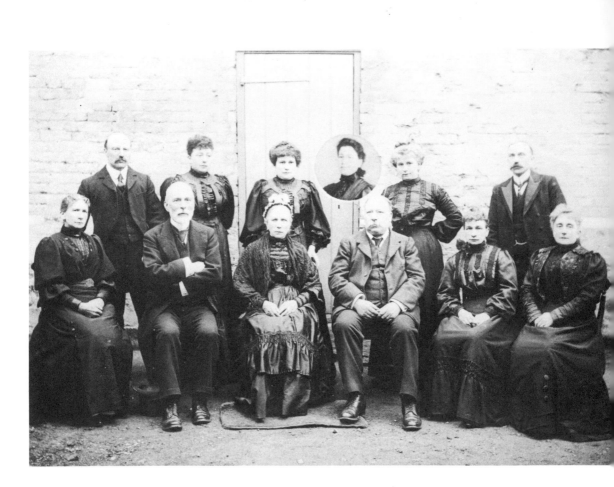

201 The well-known Walden family of Pitstow. About 1907, Elizabeth, daughter of Nathan Thurgood and Selina Pitstow, died and after her funeral, attended by all the family, a picture was taken, a likeness of Elizabeth being inserted.

Mr Pitstow, Senior, licensee of the *Eight Bells*, Bridge End, had died 25 September 1884, aged 58. Selina, his widow, continued there for a time, then moved to take over the *Cross Keys* where she died in 1911. She was succeeded by her daugher Mrs Priscilla Griggs. 'Nathan Pitstow, Walden, Publican' was admitted a member of Abbey Lane Church on 30 January 1852. *Standing, left to right:* Ernest Alfred; Annie (Mrs A. F. James); Priscilla (Mrs Griggs); Elizabeth (in circle); Alice; Herbert. *Seated:* Rosetta; Nathan John; Mrs Selina Pitstow; Frederick; Sarah Ann (Mrs Portway); Selina. (There had been another daughter who died aged 5.)

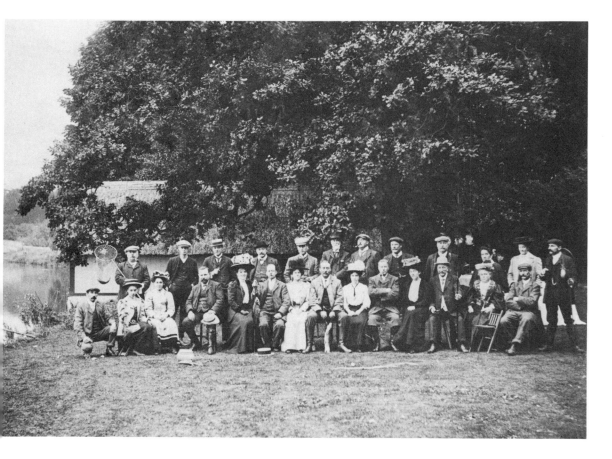

202 Saffron Walden Anglers Club taken by the Boat House at Shortgrove *circa* 1908. *Back row, left to right:* T. E. Barcham (grocer), Isaac Marking (butcher), Joseph Wright (motor car agent), ?, S. B. Donald (solicitor), Vicar of Little Sampford, J. S. W. Leverett (grocer, etc), A. E. Hearn (superintendent Isolation Hospital), – Barnes (Conservative Club), ?, ?, Wm Windwood (hairdresser). *Front row:* Julius Green (builder), ?, Miss A. Barnes, Ernest Street (draper), Miss Mabel Palmer, W. Fountain (watchmaker), Mrs Fountain, Frank Hardwick (fishmonger), Miss Fountain, Gray Palmer (clothier), Mrs F. Hardwick, George H. Archer (painter), Mrs Hearn, Tom Green (builder).

203 Friendly Societies' Athletic Sports in the Temple Park on August Bank Holidays in aid of the General Hospital. This picture would have been taken a little before 1914, for the Sports did not survive the 1914–18 War.

The Committee consisted of: Walter Parish, Herbert H. Stacey, Jim Wright and Fred Green (standing), Fred J. Taylor, Arthur Shepherd, Joseph Perry.

The articles hanging on the fence in the background are interesting because they are things one doesn't see today. They are paraffin lamps. The half-dozen cone-shaped tins held the oil. The end one shows a funnel stuck in the top of one. At the bottom of the cone was a tap which controlled the flow of paraffin down a metal tube which curved at the bottom to hold a burner. The lamp served the dual purpose of providing heat or light or both. They were commonly used in the winter months on the stalls in the Market Place but in the Park in August they were used to hang along the route from the Temple where the sports were held, to Abbey Lane Park Gates, giving light to guide the way home in the dark after the fireworks display and the 'moving pictures'. These old flare lamps were useful, but were dirty and smelly and of course the naked flame was dangerous.

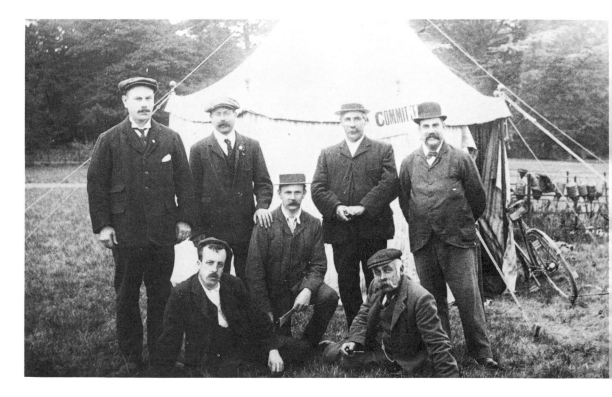

204 The Drum and Bugle Band of B Coy 3/2nd Volunteer Battalion, Essex Regiment, 1914–18 War. This picture was taken in September 1917.

Mr George Percy Horton (Asst Adjutant) went amongst the farmers and others in the Market and on the Corn Exchange and successfully appealed for subscriptions to buy drums and bugles to form a band. Alfred Pitstow (ex-Boer War) was made bandmaster and he taught us to roll and beat our drums. Sergeant Arthur Evenett, a member of the Town Band (as was Alfred Pitstow) taught the buglers. Tommy Lacey (Town Band's Bass Drummer) had the 'big drum'. During the week we practised in a shooting-range I think it was, at the back of 86 High Street, which was the Territorial's Headquarters and, for the duration of the war, the Recruiting Office. By the time we boys were got together, the volunteers had passed through the drilling stage and were engaged in the more serious training in firing their rifles. On Sundays, therefore, the band usually marched with the Company from the top of High Street to the shooting butts off the Newport Road beyond the Fulfen in the direction of Thieves Corner. The butts were frequently used by the volunteers in pre-1914 days. Old Ordnance Maps mark the butts showing all the various measured distances of the firing banks from the targets set in a deep chalk-pit cut in the side of the rising land there.

While the volunteers did their rifle practise, the band practised out of the way in the Fulfen. As we progressed, Alfred Pitstow wrote simple marches to play on the march back from the butts. We were only 14 or 15 and Alfred (whose two boys Reg and Herbert were drummers) never allowed us to bring ridicule on the Company by heading the parade trying to play marches too difficult for us. Cyril Day, the leading drummer, later played a side-drum in the Town Band and after the war he joined a Regular Army band to play a side-drum there.

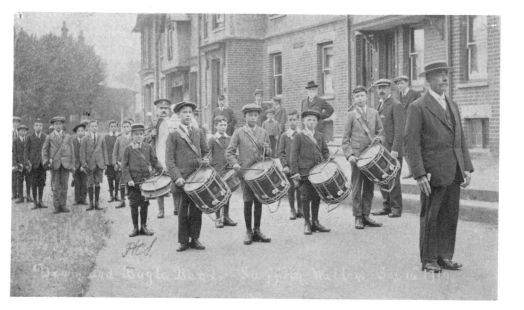

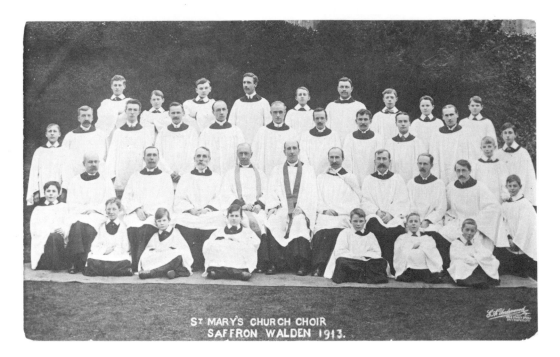

205 The Parish Church Choir, *circa* 1913. *Back:* *Billy *(Mop)* Whitehead: *Len Pitstow; Sid Newman; C. Dudley Bright (sanitary inspector); Leslie Bewers; Tom Marshall; Alf Housden; Charles Hailstone; Ronald Newman. *Second row:* –Day; ? W. E. New; H. M. Cattell; Capt P. A. Hunt; T. A. Barrett; Harry Cox; Harold Whitehead; Stan *(Marley)* Day; – Johnson (Church Street); *Charlie Shepherd; Ray Turner. *Third row:* Harold Evenett; C. H. Youngman; H. B. Jeffrey; Jasper Prime; Rev G. F. Hart; Canon J. T. Steele; Dr H. Mahon (organist and choirmaster); H. L. C. Pountney; Arthur Shepherd; G. E. Martin; Douglas Meekings. *Front:* George Burton; – Nichol; – Nichol; (two brothers from *Rose and Crown*); Teddy Shepherd; *Cyril Day; ? .

*The only known survivors 13 January 1980

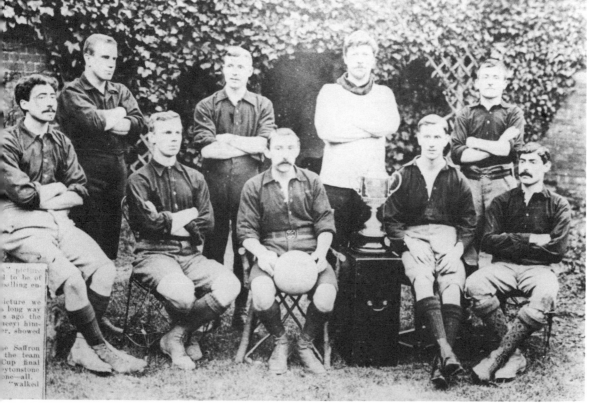

206 Saffron Walden Town Football Club 1897 – Winners of the Essex Junior Cup. The Town played Leytonstone in the first game and drew 1–1. In the replay, Walden 'walked away' with the cup a 6–1 win; *Back row;* The Rev W. E. Drinkwater (Curate), IR; A. E. Whitehead (*Sun Inn*, Church Street), RHB; Arthur Smith (Headmaster, National School), Goal; Tom Lacey, LHB; *Front row;* J. Debnam, OR; F. W. Dell, (Friends' Schoolmaster), CF; Julius Green, Back (Capt); Sidney F. Womack (Boys' British Schoolmaster), OL; Albert E. Housden, Back. *Absent from photograph:* A. Hicks (Friends' School), CHB; and E. B. Shine (Grammar School), IL.

207 Essex Junior Cup Finalists 1925–26. Cup Final played on Easter Monday, 5 April 1926, on the ground of Crittalls' Athletic Club, Cressing Road, Braintree – Saffron Walden Town v Rainham Athletic. Walden lost 2 goals to 1.

Walden's Team – *Back:* Fred (*Shrab*) Bacon; Percy (*Gamma*) Wright; Frank Hurry; Cecil Sillett; Frank Cornwell; Arthur Sell. *Seated:* K. Boyton (Barclays Bank); Albert Adams; Mr William Adams (Town Clerk), President; Herbert Lewis (Secretary); George (*Rock*) Flack; Cliff Stacey; Percy Andrews.

Rainham Athletic were finalists for Romford Charity Cup; Barking Hospital Cup; semi-finalists Grays COT Cup; leaders, South Essex League – Div II. This was their first year in Final.

Walden reached the Final of this Competition in 1894/95; 1908/09 and won the Cup in 1896/97.

At this time there were few Senior Football Clubs in Essex – Clapton; Leyton; Romford; Leytonstone; Barking were about all I think. All other clubs played 'Junior' football. And it was strictly amateur and no nonsense!

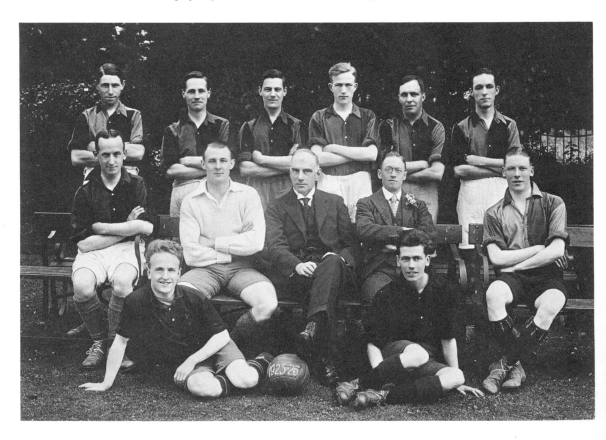

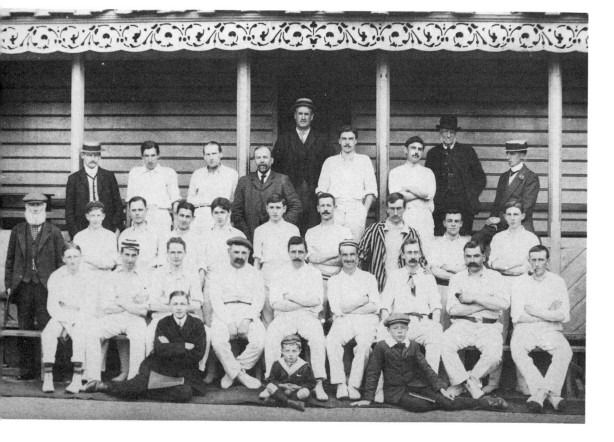

208 Saffron Walden Cricket Club. The Town Cricket Club was established in 1859 but C. B. Rowntree in *Walden Cricket* writes that on 10 August 1812, 'Eleven Gentlemen of Saffron Walden played eleven Gentlemen of Cambridge, and lost. A week later a return match was played at Walden and Cambridge won again. Each match was played for a stake of 100 guineas, so Walden lost £210 in the space of 8 days'. Rowntree does not say the match was played on the Common, but I think we can assume it was. Certainly Walden played Bishop's Stortford on Walden Common on 11 July 1837, 'the match began at 10 am lasted till 7 pm, Alfred Adams scoring 279'.

The pavilion many of us remember on the Common, was built by Wm Bell in 1871 for £150 10s. It was dismantled, moved and re-erected on the cricket ground at the Memorial Playing Fields about 1954.

I suppose all BBS boys of my generation will remember the Annual Old Boys' Match. The above is the one played 4 July 1912. *Back:* H. M. Cattell, R. A. Strong, O. B. Johnson, H. Hayes, groundsman Sid Foster, Bert Sapsford, C. Richardson, Peter Wedd, (Saddler, father of Fred), Bert Brooks. *Centre:* J. Mallion, *Billy Guy, C. G. Wood, H. M. Housden, Bert Evenett, H. (*Cutter*) Clark, C. S. Reed, E. H. Cro, Frank C. Coe, Stan Bewers. *Seated:* Stanley Adams, Herbert (*Drummer*) Wyatt, Charles Withers, Charlie Downham, H. Player, Fred (*Bonner*) Wedd, Arthur Newman, H. R. (*Tom*) Downham, Percy Cro. *Front:* Alf (*Tuck*) Penning, Phil Ketteridge, Alfred Housden

*Lost his life in the 1914–18 War when his ship was sunk at sea. Son of newsagent, Cross Street (see plate 94).

209 Tennis Club, *circa* 1912. The courts were in Station Street opposite the goods station. A study of the photograph suggests to me that it was the site of the Building Material Supply Co at the corner of Station Street and Station Road, the building in the background being the goods shed.

Persons known in the picture – *Standing, left to right:* 2. Mrs W. E. Hart, 3. Miss Edie Ramsey, 4. Miss Ethel Ramsey, (married W. G. Palmer). *Centre:* Miss Marjorie Hart. *Front:* 1. Ralph Dix, 2. Mrs Julius Green, 3. Bernard Choppen (still alive in Calgary, Canada).

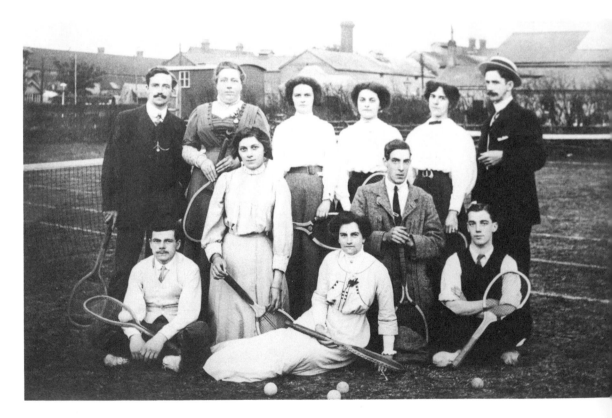

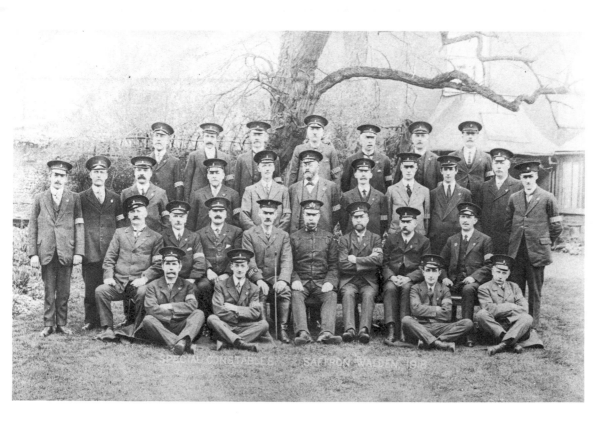

210 Walden's Special Constables in World War I. *Back row:* J. B. Burton, H. Peasgood, C. E. Spurge, H. L. Pountney, W. E. Guy, H. H. Turner, A. E. Whitehead. *Standing:* C. Richardson, H. Burton, R. E. Selves, H. Hayes, A. H. Forbes, J. S. W. Leverett, Guy Maynard, T. W. Barrett, R. A. Strong, Arthur J. Smith, J. McCaskie. *Seated:* J. W. White, J. Green, H. (*Tom*) Downham, J. W. Pateman, Supt J. E. Boyce, David Miller, F. Bell, J. R. Stewart. *Front:* Wm Freeman, Sam Harris, J. Fulger, E. A. Barnard. Taken in photographer E. A. Underwood's garden by his studio in Gold Street in 1918.

Mr C. B. Rowntree was also a Special Constable during the war, for he gave me his truncheon, which I still have. I could never imagine him using it!

211 Essex Detachment 41 Red Cross, taken at Walden Place Red Cross Hospital, 1916. *Back row:* A. G. Clay, Chas Reed, A. L. Francis, Frank Wilkerson, G. J. Bowtle, Walter Pettitt, Ernest Robinson, Arthur Green. *Second row:* Sid Newman, Percy Jarwood, ? , Chas Bradford, Edgar Miller, Harold White, ? , Stan Butt, Bert Evenett. *Third row:* Leslie Adams, Leslie Bewers, Arthur Newman, P. J. Scotney, J. S. W. Leverett, Dr J. P. Atkinson Jnr. (Commandant), Isaac Marking, Julius Green, George Wyatt, Stan Shelley. *Front:* Harry Cox, Billy Green, Albert Dew, Stacey Dyer.

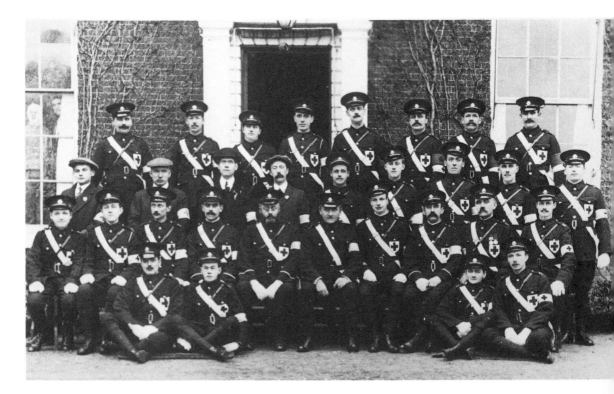

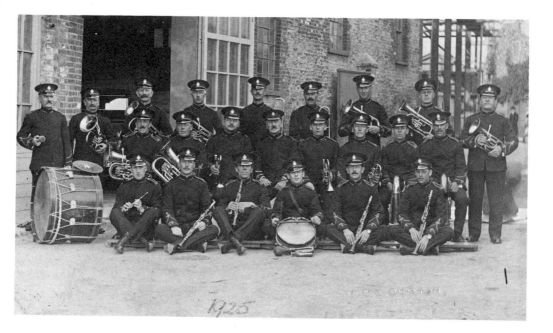

212 The Town Band. Taken in Raynham's Yard in High Street. The Bandroom was in the former Scout Headquarters on the first floor above where the band is grouped.

The picture shows the steel girders being erected at the High Street end of the brewery, to provide a motor showroom (see plate 109). The showroom covered the brewery yard behind a front brick wall with large double gates at each end for 'in' and 'out' traffic. The openings in the rear wall of the showroom were actually the loading bay for the drays and large wagons. The wagons stayed in the yard overnight. The horses were established behind what is now the *Saffron Hotel*. *Back:* Tom Lacey, Wm Badman, Chas Mallion, Alf Copping, Frank Champ, Albert Housden, Arthur Martin, Walter Pettitt, Walter Evenett. *Centre:* Fred Housden, Arthur Evenett, Arthur Badman, Ernest Pitstow (Bandmaster), Bert Evenett, Alf Holland, Cyril Auger, Chas Cornell. *Front:* Len Pitstow, Percy Freeman, Cecil Evenett, Cyril Day, Bill Stebbings, Henry Day.

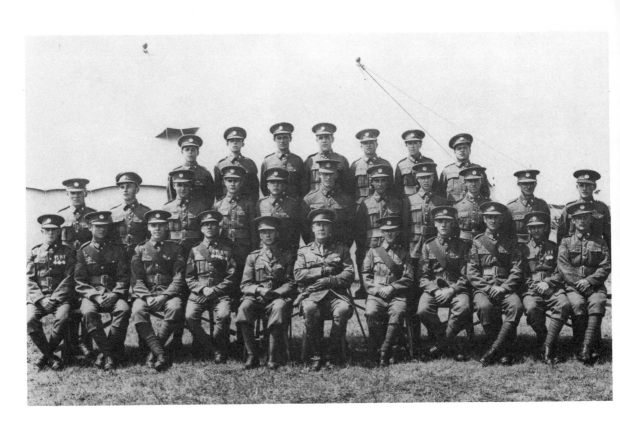

213 Walden's Territorials about 1935, taken before Morrison J. Wootton joined as a Lieutenant. Wootton joined the staff of the Borough Council to assist the Borough Engineer (H. A. Cook) in designing and building the houses in Little Walden Road to re-house the many people displaced as a result of the Council's slum clearance programme. I would think Wootton took his commission about 1937–38. He was badly wounded and died in Italy.

Back row: G. Gypps, C. Thurgood, Bert King, J. Drane (from Heydon), Heydon, ? , C. J. Reynolds. *Second row:* L. Herbert, A. King, ? , C. Lowe, *Alec Stock, – Stone, ? , †H. Ketteridge, C. Potts, W. Banks. *Third row:* Cpl F. Mason, Sgt Philip Badman, Sgt Albert W. Mummery, Sgt W. Chapman, Lieut Frank Barrett, Capt H. T. Myhill, CQMS Percy Sutton, Sgt Alf H. Mummery, Sgt Harrison (*Jack*) Sayer, Cpl C. Heydon, Cpl W. Lambert.

My recollection is that Mr Harry Myhill held the rank of Major at the time the age-limit obliged him to retire. He thought the world of his boys and continued in the Service but as a Captain. It was said when War broke out in 1939 that Capt Myhill wanted very much to be mobilised with his boys, but his age prevented it.

*1939–45 War – made prisoner.
†1939–45 War – killed.

214   1st Saffron Walden B-P Scouts, *circa* 1930. *Back row:* Cecil King, (*Nobby*) Player, Frank Chapman, Bill Clarke, Frank Sutton, Joey Taylor, Wally Everett (ASM), Bill Cowell, Jack Snow (troop leader), Eric Rumble, W. A. Mackrow (Rover Mate), Geo Lofts, Jack Swan, Dick Bird, Bill Johnson, A. (*Sandy*) Geary, Peter Housden. *Centre row:* Jim Banks, Joe Banks, George Sutton, Albert Stock, Doug Pike, Alf Sutton (SM), Stan Sillett, Cliff Stacey (CM and group secretary), Philip Badman, Cyril Edwards, Cecil Cox, Charlie Perry, Hugh Beattie, David Waters. *Wolf cubs in front:* Don Clarke, Gerald Golby, Dennis Cox, Fred White, Jack Hawkey, Micky Waters, – Clements, Montagu Shield.

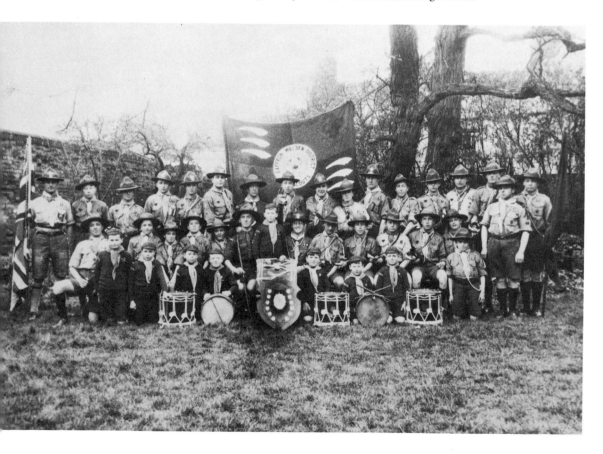

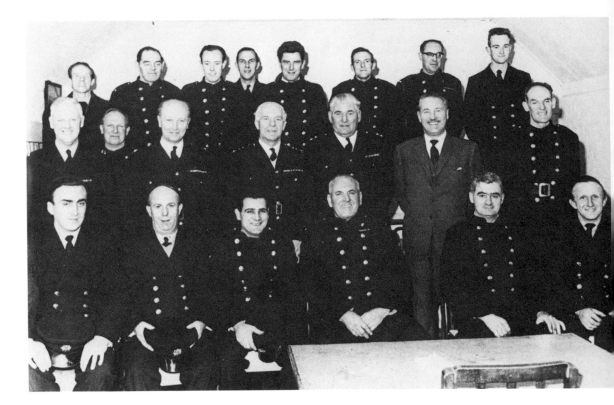

215 Fire Brigade, 1965. The Chairman of the County Fire Brigade Committee (A. H. Wright) and County Chief Fire Officer (E. Ellis) meet with the Brigade to say goodbye to Station Officer Len Crickmore, BEM, on his retirement, December 1965, after 27 years' service.

It was in 1945 that Len received from King George VI the British Empire Medal for his action when an ammunition dump exploded at Great Chesterford shortly before D-Day in June 1944.

Back: Louis Brown, Albert Mummery, Reg Burton, Angus Turnbull, Tom Cook, Frank Woodhouse, Fred Dane, Chris Payne. *Centre:* Eric Ray, Bill Sell, ? , County Chief Fire Officer E. Ellis, Len C. Crickmore, Chairman M. A. H. Wright, Ron Green. *Front:* Barry Vincent, Bob Howlett, Billy Vella, Joe Sayer, – Gibson, Jimmy Jones.

216 Fire Brigade, 1931. *On engine:* Engineer J. A. Choppen, Herbert Day, Cliff Choppen, Dick Selves Jnr, Frank Ketteridge. *Standing:* Chief Officer Clem Miller, Second Officer Arthur J. Dix, Foreman Herbert (*Drummer*) Wyatt, Hubert Bell, Teddy Worley, Dick Selves Snr.

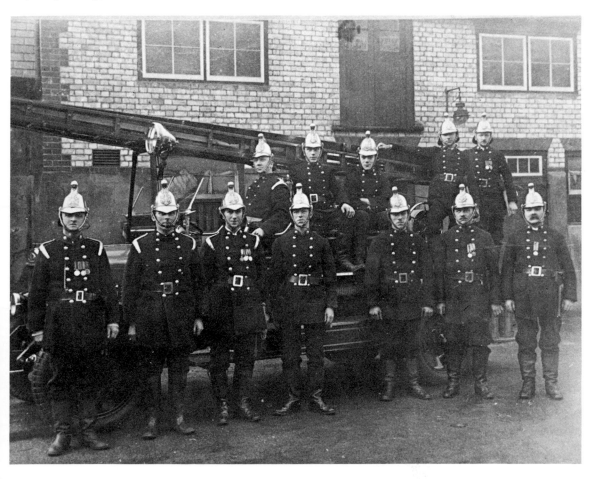

217 Saffron Bloom Lodge of Oddfellows, *circa* 1924. *Back row, left to right:* Frank Champ, Alfred Pitstow, Arthur G. Stacey, Fred J. Pitstow, Stanley Brewers, Walter Parish, John Adams. *Seated:* Sammy Legerton, Harold Cattell, Wm Green, R. A. Williams, Ernest A. Pitstow, H. B. Jeffrey, Jos Prime. *Front:* Stanley G. Butt, Arthur Newman, Percy Freeman.

At the time I was initiated into the adult Lodge, meetings were held at *The Hoops*; later the Lodge met in the Central Hall.

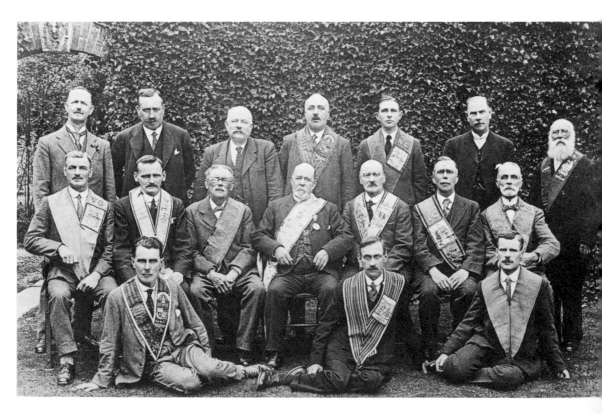

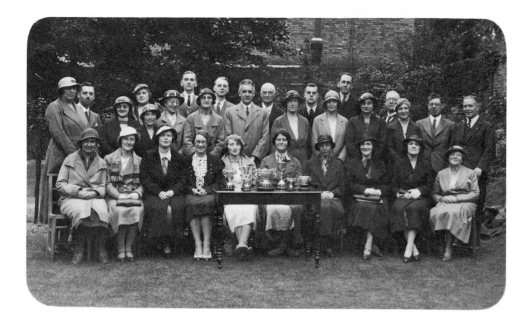

218 Saffron Walden Musical Society, *circa* 1935. *Standing – left to right:* Marjorie Hart, Owen Jones, Gladys Bloom, Mrs Engelmann, Daisy Burton, – Cunningham, Ken Choppen, Mrs White, Phillip Andrews, Louis Jeeves (Conductor), T. A. Barrett, Mrs Bert Searle, Frank Choppen, Miss F. E. Clapham, Len Darkins, Pat Ridgwell, Algy Choppen, ? , S. F. Richardson, Loftus Cox. *Seated:* Beth Titchmarsh, Gladys Harris, Betty Wandless, Nancy Stephenson, Doreen Moore, Mrs Helen Radley, Miss Lucy L. Wilkes, Mrs Choppen, Gladys Choppen, Mrs Cox.

219   Saffron Walden Male Voice Choir, *circa* 1935.
Back row – left to right:

| F. Housden | C. Farnham | F. Bunting | L. S. Darkins | E. J. Turnbull | W. O. Jones | S. F. Richardson |

Front row – left to right:

| A. W. Overall | L. Sillett | A. C. Shepherd | L. Jeeves | L. Pitstow | T. A. Dewing | H. C. Stacey |

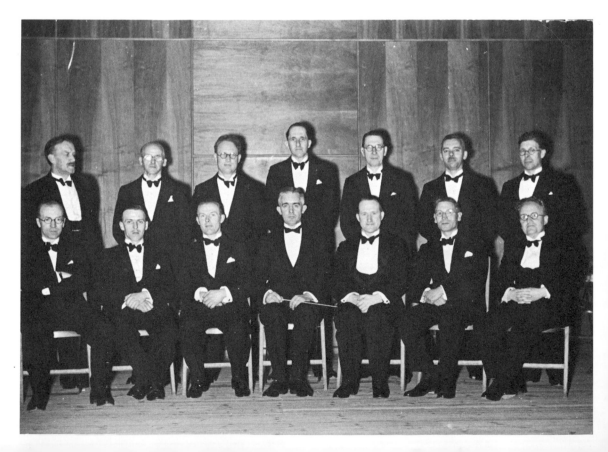

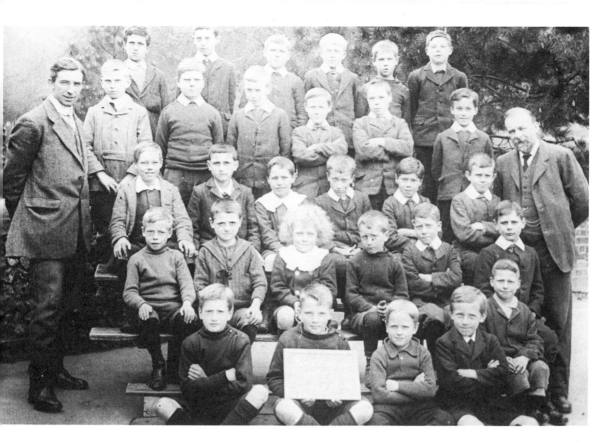

220 Boys' British School, 1912. Group 4 – Standard 5, the 10-year-olds. *Back row:* Cyril Salmon, Ernest Westwood, Tom Freeman, Duke Housden, Archie Regelous, Doug Skillings. *Second row:* Percy Baynes, T. H. Waterhouse, Willie Pinner, Frank Harris, Charlie Richardson, ? . *Third row:* Eddie Clark, Tom Sayer, Percy Wright, Dick Graves, Henry Housden, ? . *Fourth row:* Joe Clark, Charlie Sayer, Eric Wright, Len Graves, Vic Bouch, Douglas Meekings. *Front:* Mr R. A. Strong, Valentine Wichello, Ted Shepherd, Cliff Stacey, Stan Sparrow, Sid Jacobs, Mr H. Hayes.

Parents, especially those with several children, had little money to spare for school photographs, so Headmaster Hayes put the boys from the same family in the group containing the eldest brother. In this group Eddie Clark, Tom Sayer, Percy (*Gamma*) Wright and Dick Graves have their younger brothers seated in front of them.

221 Boys' British School Sports Team, 1937. *Back:* R. A. Strong, T. A. Dewing, Miss F. Ashford, Frank L. Scotford, J. P. Elsden (Headmaster). *Centre:* *A. J. Auger, *Norman Peploe, Albert Ridgwell, E. Howard, Eric Freeman. *Front:* ? Barnes, Cecil Roberts, Norman Goddard, Douglas Coe, Roy Braybrooke, Geoff Seeley.

　*Another picture names these first two boys John Thorn and Bob Peploe.

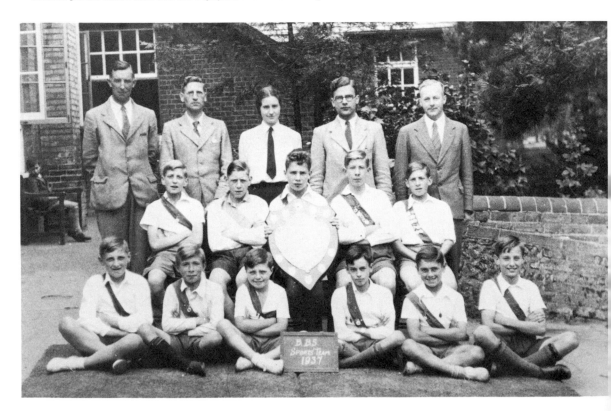

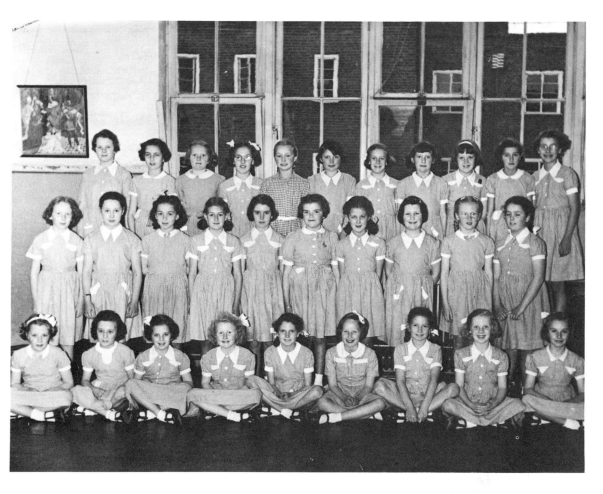

222 South Road School Music Festival, May 1954. *Back:* Janice Rushmer, Valerie Macnamara, Penny Major, Jean Banks, ? , Katherine Hopkinson, Enid Housden, Kathleen Baker, ? , Marlene Howlett, Hazell Randle. *Centre:* Sally Hudson, Maureen Harper, ? , Denise Riley, Patricia Ashman, Brenda Reed, Hazel Hare, Diane Elliott, Christine Holme, Judith Britton. *Front:* Sheila Startup, ? , Iris Stock, Elizabeth Faircloth, Elizabeth Roberts, Susan Beck, Margaret Neville, Janice Ray, Carol Sillett.

223 South Road Infants' School. Retirement of Mrs Evelyn Downham (*née* Choppen) as a teacher at the South Road Infants' School from 1939 to 1965 and at R. A. Butler Infants' School from 1965 to 1970. Taken at Mrs Downham's retirement party. *Standing left to right:* Mrs E. Jones, Mrs M. Savage (School Sec), Miss W. Reeve, Mrs Selby, Mrs Reid, Miss M. Turnbull, Mrs B. Bates, Miss D. Hurworth (Headmistress), Mrs B. Nichol, Mrs Joan Reed (Evelyn's daughter), Mrs Meg Reed, Mrs Guilbert, Mrs Floyd, Mrs Betty Harlock, Miss E. Bruton, Miss E. Harper, Mrs Vera Edwards, Mrs Flitton. *Seated;* Mrs Anne Caroll, Mrs Maud Scotford (*née* Farringdon) 1929–41, Mrs Evelyn Downham, Mrs Pat Stacey (*née* Ridgwell) 1930–36, 1956–69.

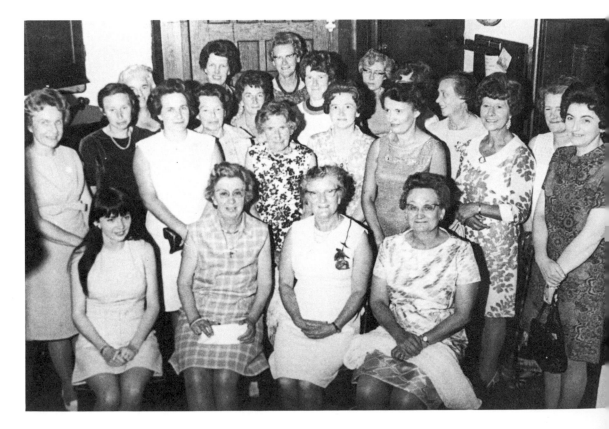

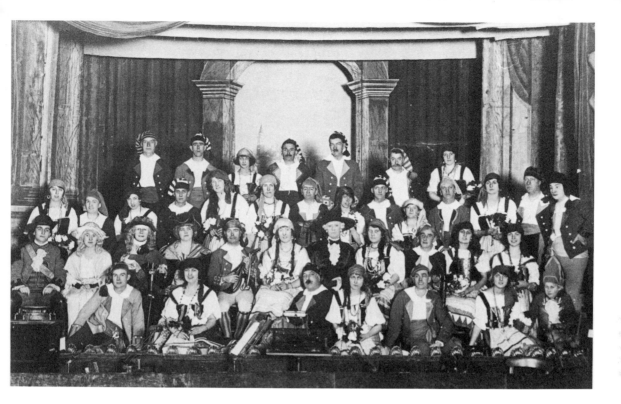

224 S.W.A.O.S. *The Gondoliers* January 1925. *Back row:* T. A. Barrett; Cyril Myhill; Gwen Barnard; Harold Whitehead; – Moore (Stationmaster), G. E. Martin; Mrs – Rate. *Third row:* Connie Dobson; Cliff Stacey; Marjorie Land; Geoffrey Barnard; May Sibley; Evelyn Guy; Tom Avery; Mrs Avery; Chas Farnham; Mrs Cox; Algy Choppen; Gladys Housden; Arthur Smith; A. C. Renner. *Second row:* C. G. Davis; Leila Welch; Louis Buck; Mrs D. Kett; Loftus Cox; Mary Guy; C. R. Gadsby; Mrs C. G. Engelmann; L. Stoneman; Enid Roberts; Gladys Pitstow. *Front row:* Charlie Shepherd; Elsie Gardner; Fred J. Pitstow; Vida Birch; Billy Green; Vera Pitstow; Cissie Leverett.

Audley End

225 Audley End Almshouses. Formerly the Walden Abbey Infirmary. Until a few years ago, these were almshouses mainly for estate employees. Now modernised and converted into the College of St Mark for retired clergy.

The College is listed as a building of historic and architectural importance. It derives its name from the original 'infirmaria' which was consecrated on St Mark's Day in 1258 by Hugo de Balsham, Bishop of Norwich. In about 1600, the buildings were re-built by the first Earl of Suffolk, who built Audley End Mansion.

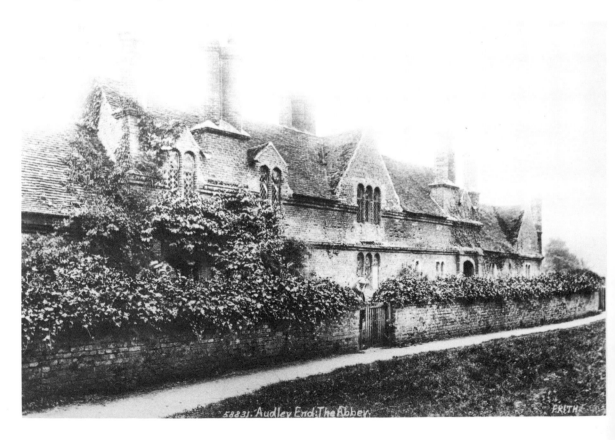

58831. Audley End. The Abbey. FRITH

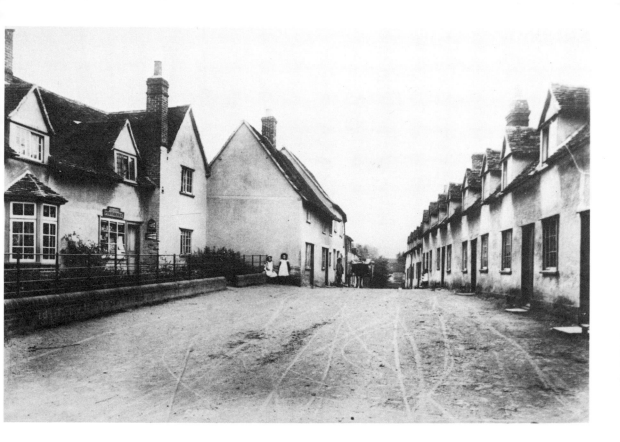

226   Audley End Village.
School and post office on the left and Mr Cowell's shop.
Pigot's Directory for 1839 gives:
Free School, Audley End – Charlotte Smith, Mistress;
Robert Cowell, Boot and Shoe Maker;
Winifred Bailey, Grocer and Tea Dealer.
1848 Directory:
Academy, Audley End – Elizabeth Conway;
Beerhouse, Boot and Shoes – Susannah Cowell;
Shopkeeper – Winifred Bailey.

Littlebury

227 Mill House, Littlebury. The home of the Dowager Lady Braybrooke when she left Audley End Mansion, *circa* 1941. R. H. Walker was at the mill in 1914 and Mrs Daniel Moore in 1900.

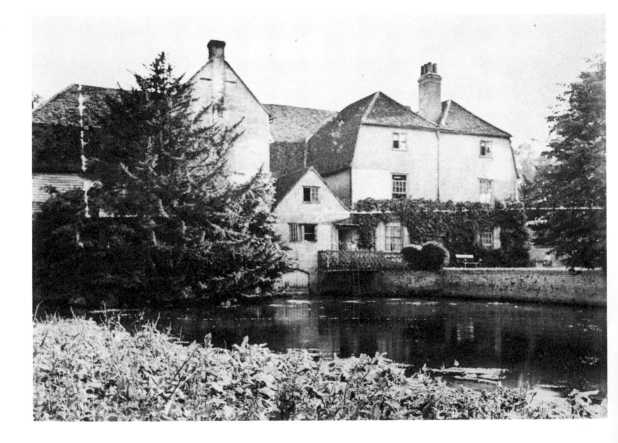

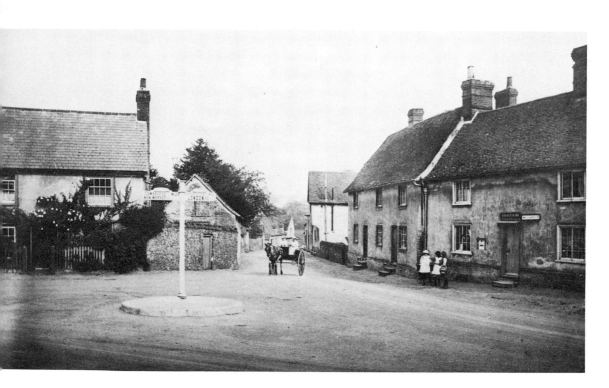

228 Littlebury, *circa* 1910. The village centre by the telegraph and post office.

Debden

229 The *Fox Inn*, Debden *circa* 1900.

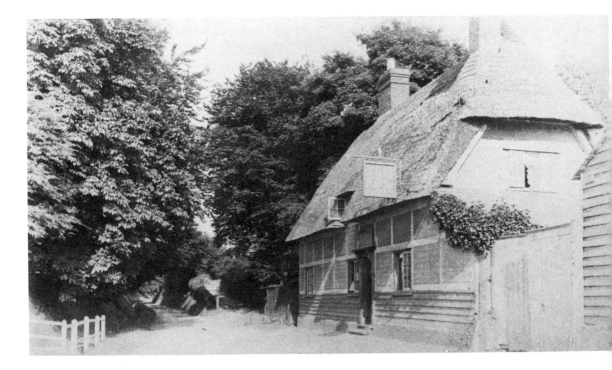

Sewards End

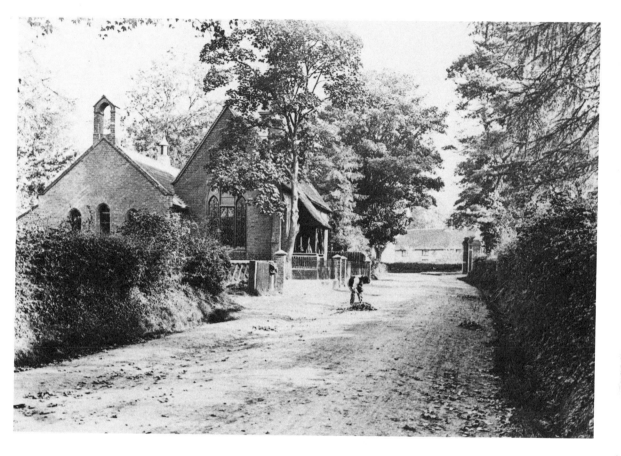

230　The church and school, *circa* 1900.

Radwinter

231 Radwinter Windmill, opposite the school, pulled down towards the end of 1920.

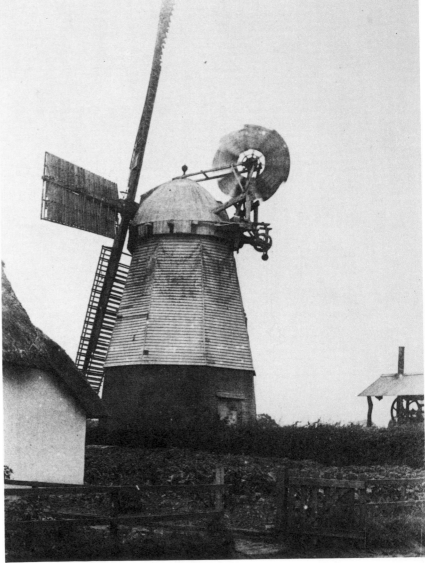